TECHNICAL
REPORT

Assessment of the Content, Design, and Dissemination of the Real Warriors Campaign

Joie D. Acosta, Laurie T. Martin, Michael P. Fisher,
Racine Harris, Robin M. Weinick

Prepared for the Office of the Secretary of Defense

RAND Center for Military Health Policy Research

A JOINT ENDEAVOR OF RAND HEALTH AND THE
RAND NATIONAL DEFENSE RESEARCH INSTITUTE

The research described in this report was prepared for the Office of the Secretary of Defense (OSD). The research was conducted jointly by the Center for Military Health Policy Research, a RAND Health program, and the Forces and Resources Policy Center, a RAND National Defense Research Institute (NDRI) program. NDRI is a federally funded research and development center sponsored by OSD, the Joint Staff, the Unified Combatant Commands, the Navy, the Marine Corps, the defense agencies, and the defense Intelligence Community under Contract W74V8H-06-C-0002.

Library of Congress Cataloging-in-Publication Data

Assessment of the content, design, and dissemination of the Real Warriors Campaign / Joie D. Acosta ... [et al.].
p. cm.
Includes bibliographical references.
ISBN 978-0-8330-6310-6 (pbk. : alk. paper)
1. Soldiers—Mental health services—United States—Evaluation. 2. United States—Armed Forces—Mental health services—Evaluation. 3. Mass media in health education—United States. I. Acosta, Joie D.

UH629.3.A77 2012
362.2086'970973—dc23

2012011679

Published 2012 by the RAND Corporation
1776 Main Street, P.O. Box 2138, Santa Monica, CA 90407-2138
1200 South Hayes Street, Arlington, VA 22202-5050
4570 Fifth Avenue, Suite 600, Pittsburgh, PA 15213-2665
RAND URL: http://www.rand.org/
To order RAND documents or to obtain additional information, contact
Distribution Services: Telephone: (310) 451-7002;
Fax: (310) 451-6915; Email: order@rand.org

Preface

An increasing number of studies and news articles have highlighted concerns about deployment-related mental health problems among military service personnel. Recognizing that barriers to obtaining mental health care were a critical issue, the Department of Defense (DoD) has implemented numerous programs designed to address issues related to mental health and psychological well-being among servicemembers and their families, including programs designed to promote resilience and reintegration of servicemembers returning from combat zones, and to support their families. The Real Warriors Campaign is one such program.

The purpose of this report is to present findings based upon an independent assessment of the content, design, and dissemination of the Real Warriors Campaign. The assessment was conducted between January and August 2011. Launched in 2009, the Real Warriors Campaign is a large-scale multimedia program designed to promote resilience, facilitate recovery, and support the reintegration of returning servicemembers, veterans, and their families. The campaign itself is fairly new; at the time of this report, there was the possibility of changes to the content or dissemination of the campaign because the contract to manage the campaign was being re-competed. Therefore, the assessment described in this report focuses on identifying which aspects of the campaign adhere to best practices for health communication campaigns and ways the campaign could improve both its content and its dissemination activities. To conduct the assessment we convened an expert panel, conducted telephone discussions with organizations that partnered with the campaign, performed a content analysis of the campaign's website, analyzed communication measures collected by the campaign, and reviewed relevant documents describing the design and development of the campaign.

The contents of this report will be of particular interest to national policymakers within the DoD and should also be useful for health policy officials within the U.S. Department of Veterans Affairs (VA), as well as policymakers in other sectors who sponsor or manage media campaigns to support mental health more generally.

This research was sponsored by the Assistant Secretary of Defense for Health Affairs and the Defense Centers of Excellence for Psychological Health and Traumatic Brain Injury (DCoE) and conducted jointly by RAND Health's Center for Military Health Policy Research and the Forces and Resources Policy Center of the RAND National Defense Research Institute (NDRI). The Center for Military Health Policy Research taps RAND expertise in both defense and health policy to conduct research for DoD, the Veterans Health Administration, and nonprofit organizations. NDRI is a federally funded research and development center sponsored by the Office of the Secretary of Defense, the Joint Staff, the Unified Combatant Commands, the Navy, the Marine Corps, the defense agencies, and the defense Intelligence Community.

For more information on the Center for Military Health Policy Research, see http://www.rand.org/multi/military.html or contact the director (contact information is provided on the web page). For more information on the RAND Forces and Resources Policy Center, see http://www.rand.org/nsrd/ndri/centers/frp.html or contact the director (contact information is provided on the web page).

Contents

Figures

Tables

Summary

Over the past decade, increasing concerns about the mental health and psychological well-being of U.S. service personnel have been well documented. Research has suggested that, as of October 2007, between 25 and 30 percent of veterans from Operation Iraqi Freedom and Operation Enduring Freedom (OIF/OEF) have reported symptoms of a mental health problem (Seal, Bertenthal, et al., 2007; Tanielian and Jaycox, 2008), and a 2011 study found that 37 percent of veterans reported suffering from post-traumatic stress (Pew Research Center, 2011). Recognizing that barriers to mental health care were a critical issue in need of further exploration, the Department of Defense (DoD) convened several task forces to assess the mental health of servicemembers and to examine the delivery of mental health care. In response to the work of these task forces, the DoD implemented numerous programs designed to address issues related to mental health, including post-traumatic stress disorder (PTSD) and psychological well-being among servicemembers and for their families.

One ongoing challenge for the DoD has been to identify and characterize the scope, nature, and effectiveness of these various and continuously evolving activities. At the request of the DoD, the RAND Corporation conducted a systematic cataloguing of all DoD-funded programs designed to address issues related to mental health, psychological well-being, and traumatic brain injury among servicemembers and their families (Weinick, Beckjord, et al., 2011). As an additional phase of this project, RAND is undertaking a limited number of evaluations of programs that hold promise for addressing the mental health needs of servicemembers and their families. The Real Warriors Campaign (RWC), a large-scale multimedia program designed to promote resilience, facilitate recovery, and support the reintegration of returning servicemembers, veterans, and their families, was selected as one such program. The RWC is operated by the Defense Centers of Excellence for Psychological Health and Traumatic Brain Injury (DCoE) via a contract with Booz Allen Hamilton.

Purpose of the Report

This report summarizes RAND's independent assessment of the design, content, and dissemination of the RWC, which was conducted between January and August 2011. The RWC is a relatively new effort, launched in 2009. This assessment was designed to do the following:

1. Document the design (goals, target populations, and core messages) and content of the RWC and how the content is disseminated to target populations.

2. Identify the strengths of the design, content, and dissemination strategies used by the RWC and which aspects of the campaign adhere to best practices for health communication campaigns.
3. Identify where DoD should target future investments or quality improvement efforts related to the RWC.

This study was designed as a preliminary assessment because the campaign itself is fairly new. Further, at the time our assessment was conducted, the contract to manage the campaign was being re-competed. Given the possibility of changes to the content or dissemination of the RWC due to the new contract, further evaluation activities would be more valuable after any potential changes to the campaign were made. Once the campaign has time to further mature in its outreach efforts and the issues we identify have been addressed, the RWC may benefit from a full-scale program evaluation. Such future evaluations should include an assessment of campaign penetration rates and detailed feedback from the target population.

Rationale for the Real Warriors Campaign

Despite efforts by both the DoD and the Department of Veterans Affairs (VA) to enhance mental health services, many servicemembers are still not regularly seeking needed care when they have mental health problems. Without appropriate treatment, these mental health problems can have a wide-ranging and negative impact on the quality of life and social, emotional, and cognitive functioning of affected servicemembers. Untreated mental health problems can also compound the costs of engaging in combat by increasing both the medical costs of treating servicemembers who delay getting treatment and the direct costs of replacing servicemembers who leave or are compelled to leave service before completing their contracts.

In 2007, a congressionally mandated task force on mental health issued several recommendations about how to improve access to and delivery of mental health care. The RWC was developed in response to Recommendation 5.1.1.1 of the 2007 Department of Defense Mental Health Task Force report (Defense Health Board Task Force on Mental Health, 2007), which stated: "The Department of Defense should implement an anti-stigma public education campaign, using evidence based techniques to provide factual information about mental disorders."

Design, Content, and Dissemination of the Real Warriors Campaign

Using the Health Belief Model (HBM)[1] as the campaign framework, RWC staff conducted literature reviews, focus groups, and in-depth interviews, as well as market analysis, to identify the threats perceived by servicemembers experiencing mental health concerns, the perceived and real motivators to taking action, the benefits and barriers to reaching out for care that exist within the military community, and the tactics that would influence behavior change. RWC staff used this information to develop and identify the target populations, campaign goals, core messages, and dissemination strategies for the campaign.

[1] The HBM is a widely used model that identifies key influences (e.g., perceptions of individual susceptibility to a health problem) that predict whether an individual will take action to address a health issue.

This research led to the identification of five relevant target populations for the campaign: active duty servicemembers, members of the Reserve and National Guard, veterans, families, and health professionals. Additionally, the RWC developed four campaign goals that map to the four constructs in the HBM:

- raising awareness about the signs and symptoms of mental health concerns
- raising awareness about the relative costs of inaction compared with action in seeking help for mental health concerns
- raising expectations for positive outcomes for seeking support or treatment
- raising awareness about the resources and services available for support and treatment.

The campaign's core messages were designed to reinforce these goals by helping servicemembers, veterans, and their families understand that they are not alone in experiencing and dealing with mental health concerns and that resources for care and treatment are available and effective.

The campaign reaches servicemembers, veterans, members of the National Guard and Reserve, families, and health care professionals through a variety of communication channels. These include the RWC website, social media, partnership activities, and conferences and events.

RAND's Independent Assessment of the Real Warriors Campaign

Methods

To conduct the assessment of the design, content, and dissemination of the RWC, we utilized six complementary methods:

1. a search of the peer-reviewed literature to identify best practices and the empirically defined characteristics and qualities of effective behavioral health media campaigns
2. an expert panel to determine the extent to which the campaign reflects current best practices in health communication campaigns
3. telephone discussions with RWC partner organizations to assess how the campaign has been disseminated and to determine partner organizations' perceptions of the campaign and its materials
4. a content analysis of the website to determine its relevance to the target populations; alignment with campaign goals; function within the campaign (e.g., educational information, resources to promote help-seeking, promotion of the RWC); and whether the content provided connections to services, additional information, or support
5. an analysis of communication measures collected by the RWC to triangulate findings from the partner discussions and expert panel
6. a document review and informal discussions with RWC staff to gather information about how the RWC was designed.

Our assessment focused primarily on campaign activities, including the development of goals, target populations, and core messages; content development; and dissemination of the content. These activities were designed by the RWC staff to influence the four constructs in the Health Belief Model (perceived susceptibility, perceived consequences, perceived benefits, and perceived barriers).

Results

Table S.1 shows the key findings from our assessment for each campaign activity.

Table S.1
Findings from the Assessment of the Real Warriors Campaign

Campaign Activity	Findings
Campaign design: Development of goals, target population, and core messages	Campaign goals were clear to experts and partner organizations but are not stated on the website or in the campaign materials. The goals of the campaign did not align as well with health professionals as with other target audiences. There are important differences within the campaign's target audiences (e.g., varying ages and races) that should be considered throughout the development of the campaign messages, materials, and dissemination strategies. The core messages of the campaign were relevant and constituted the right messages for the campaign; however, as with the campaign goals, the core messages of the campaign are not stated clearly anywhere on the website.
Content development	The video profiles containing personal stories of servicemembers struggling with mental health problems were the "heart" of the campaign and were consistently described as "compelling" by both the expert panelists and partner organizations. Partners and expert panelists indicated that there was too much content on the website, describing it as "overly dense" and causing "information overload," and remarked that the long lists of links, resources, and materials did not provide enough direction to users on how to prioritize the information. Much of the website content and many of the most frequently viewed articles were not directly relevant to any of the campaign goals. Coverage across target populations was uneven, with more of the website and materials focusing on the active duty population. Several of the links to resources and other materials were not working and some of the expert panelists expressed concern that the content of the website was quickly becoming outdated.
Dissemination of content	While the RWC website is a potentially helpful tool for reaching the campaign's target audiences, panelists felt that key components of the site should be better highlighted and suggested technological solutions to increase website navigability and interactivity. Although most of the campaign's social media tools are viewed as useful by its partners and are growing in popularity among target audiences, utilization is still limited and some of these dissemination channels appear to be more useful than others. Although not all partner organizations are actively engaged in disseminating the campaign, 59 percent disseminate campaign information materials and resources through articles, news briefs, e-blasts, e-newsletters, social media, or blogs, or at venues such as conferences, events, offices, or clinics. Approximately two-thirds of the partners we spoke with made suggestions for improvement of the campaign's partnership program.
Use of research and ongoing monitoring	RWC staff reported using both research and stakeholder analysis as the basis for developing campaign messages and tactics. Although the campaign collects and reports a range of communication metrics, the information from these metrics was not being used to help guide strategic decisions about the campaign. Beyond the communication metrics described above, the RWC does not conduct any ongoing process or outcome evaluation. Both partner organizations and the expert panelists suggested that the RWC needs to regularly seek feedback on its website and materials and on the relevance of the messages it is disseminating. The RWC has not conducted any usability testing of the website since the website was launched.

Limitations of Our Assessment

Our evaluation was limited in scope to an assessment of campaign activities. We focused our efforts on the core elements of the campaign: its goals, target populations, and core messages; the ways in which those elements were executed to create meaningful, relevant, and actionable campaign materials; and the methods and strategies used by the campaign to disseminate those messages. While this approach provided important insight into the strengths and opportunities for improving campaign activities, it does not provide information on the effectiveness of the campaign in achieving short-term or intermediate outcomes such as gains in knowledge or changes in perceptions related to help-seeking. Another limitation of our evaluation is that we were not able to collect data from target audiences due to time, budgetary, and logistical constraints. Finally, we did not assess the campaign's penetration rates.

Recommendations to Improve Future Design, Content, and Dissemination of the Real Warriors Campaign

Below, we summarize our recommendations to improve the design, content, and dissemination of the RWC, as well as our recommendations for improving the RWC's use of research and evaluation. We recognize that the RWC may not be able to implement all of these recommendations, but we offer them as ideas for consideration as the RWC is being continually improved and refined. It is also possible that the awareness of an external assessment and the process of re-competing the RWC contract may have already prompted some changes in the campaign between the time of our assessment and publication of this report. As a result, some of the recommendations may have been addressed. Therefore, our recommendations should be considered in light of any recent changes to the campaign.

Based on our assessment, we recommend the following changes to the RWC design and content that could improve the effectiveness of the RWC:

- Clearly state the goals and core messages of the RWC on the website.
- Review content and links on the website to ensure that they are still current.
- Streamline existing website content to ensure that it aligns with goals and key messages.
- Base the development of new goals and messages on findings from objective data sources, such as the Mental Health Advisory Team survey.
- Optimize the web layout of existing content.
- Improve the tailoring of website content to specific target populations.

Several recommendations for how the RWC can improve the reach and effectiveness of its dissemination emerged from our findings:

- Enhance and grow the social media channels that are the most effective.
- Become more proactive in the dissemination of information.
- Utilize partners more effectively.

To improve the RWC's ability to conduct continuous quality improvement, monitor progress, and assess its short- and long-term impacts, we recommend that the RWC do the following:

- Solicit regular feedback from partners.
- Engage in regular usability testing of the website.
- Convene an ongoing expert or advisory panel to help the campaign stay current and highlight key issues.
- Use improved communication metrics to conduct ongoing monitoring.
- Conduct ongoing evaluation to assess whether the campaign is meeting its short- and long-term goals.

Our assessment of the RWC design, content, and dissemination strategies suggests that the RWC shows promise in its ability to reach the intended target audiences and achieve its goals. We found that the RWC is generally adhering to best practices for health communication campaigns. However, to be responsive to the evolving needs of the military community, media campaigns like the RWC will need to invest in mechanisms that allow them to be nimble. The RWC should consider

- clearly communicating the goals of the campaign on its website and in its materials so that those goals are evident to users and partner organizations, particularly if they change over time
- more effectively leveraging the existing network of partner organizations
- conducting ongoing research and regular usability testing.

Acknowledgments

We gratefully acknowledge the assistance of the Real Warriors Campaign staff and administrators who provided support during the assessment process: Julie Hughes, Dana Stirk, and Ruth Seeley from Booz Allen Hamilton; and Catherine Haight from the Defense Centers of Excellence for Psychological Health and Traumatic Brain Injury. We also thank Kate Barker for the administrative support she provided preparing this document. In addition, we thank our project monitor at the Defense Centers of Excellence for Psychological Health and Traumatic Brain Injury, Col Christopher Robinson, CAPT Dayami Liebenguth, and Dr. Richard Sechrest, for their support of our work. We also appreciate the valuable insights we received from Lisa Meredith and Patrick Corrigan. Their constructive critiques were addressed as part of RAND's rigorous quality assurance process to improve the quality of this report. Finally, we thank the expert panel, convened as part of the evaluation, for sharing their time and feedback: Cynthia Bauer, Rebecca Collins, Howard Goldman, Harold Kudler, Deborah Leiter, Brett Litz, Shelley MacDermid, John Parrish, Aaron Rochlen, and Nancy Vineburgh.

Abbreviations

DAF	data abstraction form
DCoE	Defense Centers of Excellence for Psychological Health and Traumatic Brain Injury
DoD	Department of Defense
HBM	Health Belief Model
LOA	Line of Action
MHAT	Mental Health Advisory Team
MHTF	mental health task force
OEF	Operation Enduring Freedom
OIF	Operation Iraqi Freedom
PSA	public service announcement
PTSD	post-traumatic stress disorder
RWC	Real Warriors Campaign
SOC	Senior Oversight Committee
TBI	traumatic brain injury
VA	Department of Veterans Affairs
VHA	Veterans Health Administration
VSO	Veterans Service Organization

CHAPTER ONE

Introduction

Since 2001, there has been increasing concern about deployment-related mental health problems and psychological well-being among U.S. service personnel. Recent research has suggested that, as of October 2007, between 25 and 30 percent of veterans from Operation Iraqi Freedom and Operation Enduring Freedom (OIF/OEF) have reported symptoms of a mental health problem (Seal, Bertenthal, et al., 2007; Tanielian and Jaycox, 2008), and a 2011 study found that 37 percent of veterans reported suffering from post-traumatic stress (Pew Research Center, 2011). The prevalence of mental health problems among servicemembers is also greater than among the general U.S. population: Fourteen percent of previously deployed servicemembers have post-traumatic stress disorder (PTSD) compared with 3.6 percent in the general population, and 14 percent have major depression compared with 6.7 percent in the general population (Tanielian and Jaycox, 2008; National Institute of Mental Health, 2010a, 2010b). Recent findings from the 2010 Joint Mental Health Advisory Team Survey also suggest that the prevalence of depression, anxiety, and acute stress among servicemembers has significantly increased since 2005.

To address this growing need, Department of Defense (DoD) leaders commissioned multiple task forces, including the DoD Independent Review Group (Independent Review Group, 2007) and two independent but complementary groups commissioned by President George W. Bush: the Task Force on Returning Global War on Terror Heroes (2007), which focused on the Department of Veterans Affairs (VA), and the President's Commission on Care for America's Returning Wounded Warriors (2007). Recognizing that barriers to care were a critical issue in need of further exploration, the DoD also convened a mental health task force (MHTF), the Defense Health Board Task Force on Mental Health (2007) to assess the mental health of servicemembers deployed for ground combat and to examine the delivery of mental health care in OEF.

Reports from these groups identified a number of gaps in the treatment and rehabilitation of returning wounded, ill, and injured servicemembers and their families, and provided recommendations for improving the treatment and support of servicemembers and their families facing issues related to mental health. In response to these reports, the Secretary of Defense and the Secretary of Veterans Affairs chartered and co-chaired a Senior Oversight Committee (SOC) to streamline, integrate, and expedite efforts of the DoD and the VA to address concerns about the processes for treatment, evaluation, and transition of wounded servicemembers. The SOC was organized around eight workgroups, known as Lines of Action (LOAs). The second LOA (LOA2) was focused on developing, coordinating, and implementing DoD policies, programs, and oversight in the areas of traumatic brain injury and mental health. Its goals were identifying strategies to improve access to care for traumatic brain injury and mental health; enhancing care quality; increasing psychological resilience; decreasing stigma; improving screening and surveillance of mental health and traumatic brain injury; enhancing transition care and support; and enhancing collaboration in research. A major outcome of the LOA2 efforts was the creation of the Defense Centers of Excellence for Psychological Health and Traumatic Brain Injury (DCoE) in October 2007.

One ongoing challenge for the DoD has been to identify and characterize the scope, nature, and effectiveness of these various and continuously evolving activities. At the request of the DoD, RAND recently completed a systematic assessment of all DoD-funded programs designed to address issues related to mental health, including PTSD, psychological well-being, and traumatic brain injury among servicemembers and their families (Weinick, Beckjord, et al., 2011). As an additional phase of this project, RAND is undertaking a limited number of evaluations of programs that hold promise for addressing the mental health needs of servicemembers and their families. The Real Warriors Campaign (RWC), a large-scale multimedia program designed to promote resilience, facilitate recovery, and support the reintegration of returning servicemembers, veterans, and their families, was selected as one such program.

Purpose of This Report

This report summarizes our independent assessment of the design, content, and dissemination of the RWC. The RWC is a relatively new effort, launched in 2009 by DCoE via a contract with Booz Allen Hamilton. The campaign's activities and its theoretical basis can be synthesized into a logic model that summarizes how the campaign activities are designed to affect help-seeking for mental health problems among current and former servicemembers. This logic model can be used to examine the effectiveness of individual components of the campaign, identifying areas of strength as well as those areas with potential opportunity for improvement. Figure 1.1 presents the logic model we developed for use in our independent assessment of the RWC activities.

Our assessment focuses on the campaign's activities: design of the campaign during which goals were developed, the target population was identified, and core messages were developed; development of content including videos, articles/educational materials, resources, hotlines, print materials, and posters; and dissemination of the content via websites, conferences, presentations, and social networks. As shown in the logic model, these activities were designed to help servicemembers feel less isolated; know more about the prevalence, signs, and symptoms of mental health problems and available resources; and improve their perception that seeking help has benefits and can be nonthreatening to servicemembers' personal and professional lives (short and intermediate outcomes). As a result, servicemembers will be motivated to seek appropriate help for mental health problems (ultimate outcome). The premise that lowering the perceived threat associated with seeking help and raising the perceived benefits will result in help-seeking behavior is consistent with the Health Belief Model (HBM), which serves as the theoretical basis for the RWC and is discussed further in Chapter Two (Henshaw and Freedman-Doan, 2009).

Although our findings may provide insight into how well the campaign activities influence short-term and intermediate outcomes, this was not an explicit focus of our assessment. This study was designed as a preliminary assessment (conducted between January and August 2011) because the campaign itself is fairly new. Further, at the time our assessment was con-

Figure 1.1
Logic Model for RAND Assessment

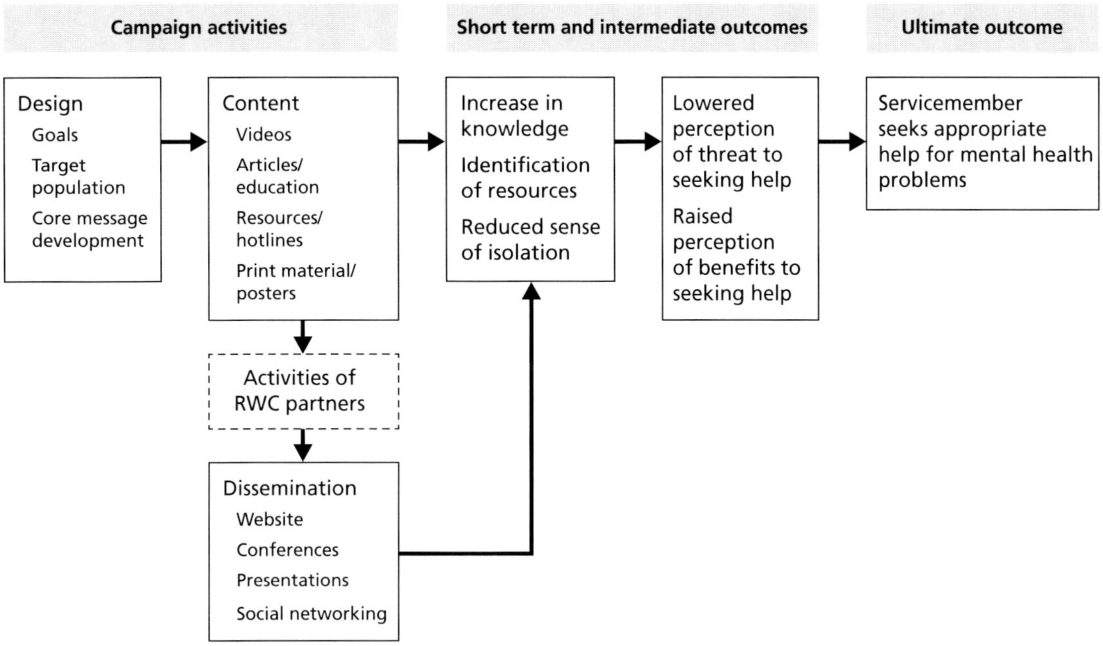

RAND *TR1176-1.1*

ducted, the contract to manage the campaign was being re-competed, suggesting that additional evaluation activities would be more valuable after management changes and any content or dissemination redesign takes place.

Once the campaign has time to further mature in its outreach efforts and the issues related to campaign design, content, and dissemination that we discuss in this report have been addressed, the RWC may benefit from a full-scale program evaluation. Such future evaluations should include an assessment of campaign penetration rates and detailed target population feedback.

Our assessment was guided by three aims:

1. Document the design (goals, target populations, and core messages) and content of the RWC and how the content is disseminated to target populations.
2. Identify the strengths of the design, content, and dissemination strategies used by the RWC and which aspects of the campaign adhere to best practices for health communication campaigns.
3. Identify where DoD should target future investments or quality improvement efforts related to the RWC.

Methods

To achieve these aims, we utilized six complementary methods: (1) a search of the peer-reviewed literature; (2) an expert panel; (3) telephone discussions with RWC partner organizations; (4) a content analysis of the RWC website; (5) an analysis of communication metrics collected by the RWC; and (6) a document review and informal discussions with RWC staff. Data collected through each of the methods helped inform different aims. Table 1.1 provides a crosswalk showing the relationship between each of the methods and the study aims. A broad summary of each method is provided below and in Appendix A. Detailed descriptions of each method are provided in Appendixes B through F.

Table 1.1
Methods Used for Each Aim

Method	Aim 1: Document design, content, and dissemination of RWC	Aim 2: Identify strengths and aspects of RWC that adhere to best practices	Aim 3: Identify areas where improvements or future investments are needed
Literature review		X	
Expert panel		X	X
Telephone discussions with partner organizations	X	X	X
Content analysis		X	X
Analysis of communication metrics		X	X
Document review and discussions with RWC staff	X	X	

Literature Review

Between January and February 2011, we conducted a search of the peer-reviewed literature to identify best practices and empirically defined characteristics and qualities of effective behavioral health media campaigns. For each article identified, we recorded lessons learned or best practices for designing, formatting, and disseminating a media campaign. These lessons learned or best practices were synthesized into a list of proposed best practices for health communication campaigns that was vetted and refined through our expert panel, discussed next. A detailed description of the literature review methods, including a summary of the literature reviewed and a list of articles, can be found in Appendix B.

Expert Panel

Between June and August 2011, we convened an expert panel to determine the extent to which the campaign reflected current best practices in health communication campaigns. The panel consisted of ten experts in five key areas:

- barriers to mental health care, including stigma
- mental health in the military (service-related PTSD, deployment psychology)
- effective media campaigns

- media campaigns for servicemembers
- psychological resilience.

Experts participated in a two-phase process to develop a checklist of best practices in health communication campaigns and then to apply a subset of items from the checklist to the RWC. During the first phase, we utilized a modified version of the RAND Appropriateness Method (Fitch, Bernstein, et al., 2001) to develop a checklist of best practices in health communication campaigns. In the second phase (August 2011), experts rated the RWC using the seven checklist items that focused on the campaign website. A list of the expert panelists and a more detailed description of their activities is included in Appendix C.

Telephone Discussions with RWC Partner Organizations

Between April and June 2011, we conducted 30-minute semistructured telephone discussions with staff at 26 of the 153 RWC partner organizations to assess how the campaign has been disseminated and to determine partner organizations' perceptions of the campaign and its materials. This included a discussion of how the organizations partner with the campaign and utilize campaign materials, as well as their perceptions of the utility and effectiveness of campaign materials. Discussions were transcribed and analyzed using standard qualitative analysis techniques, described further in Appendix D. A list of partner organizations can also be found in Appendix D.

Content Analysis of the RWC Website

In May 2011, RAND staff conducted an analysis of all content on the RWC website, including the articles, campaign dissemination materials, and video and radio public-service announcements. The content of the website was reviewed to determine its relevance to the target populations; alignment with campaign goals; function within the campaign (e.g., educational information, resources to promote help-seeking, promotion of the RWC); and whether the content provided connections to services, additional information, or support. A summary of the content reviewed and a more detailed description of the review process are included in Appendix E.

Analysis of RWC Communication Measures

In January 2011, we requested a limited number of communication measures from the RWC as an additional source of data and used these metrics to triangulate findings from the partner discussions and expert panel. These included the following:

- **Website.** The number of unique visitors to the website; number of page views; the number of times articles, videos, and public service announcements (PSAs) are viewed; the amount of time people spend on the website; popular content; the number of DoD, VA, or community resources that are accessed, and which specific resources are accessed; and websites from which viewers of the RWC are referred
- **Media Relations.** The number of times PSAs have aired; the tone and location of coverage; and the number of media impressions garnered from print, broadcast, and online media coverage on DoD and civilian outlets

- **Social Media.** The number and types of individuals connecting with the campaign and sharing information with their networks through Facebook, Twitter, YouTube, message boards, and other social networking tools
- **Outreach.** The number of partnering organizations that include campaign information in their publications; the number and names of external entities ordering such campaign materials as brochures, posters, and other hard copy materials; the number of campaign materials disseminated; and the number of individuals that RWC materials reach when attending conferences
- **Multimedia.** The number of times each video profile, or story of a servicemember who has sought help, has been viewed and the number and types of organizations downloading and using the profiles.

These metrics were analyzed by RAND staff to determine how the RWC materials are being disseminated, who is utilizing the RWC website, and how it is being utilized. This analysis is described in greater detail in Appendix F.

Document Review and Discussions with RWC Staff

We also reviewed background documents and held discussions with RWC staff to gather information about how the RWC was designed. Chapter Two provides an overview of design and dissemination of the RWC and Chapter Three summarizes findings from these data sources.

Organization of This Report

Chapter Two describes the rationale, content, and design, of the RWC and how the campaign is disseminated to target populations (Aim 1). Chapter Three provides a detailed description of our assessment of the RWC activities, including the strengths of the campaign and areas where the campaign adheres to best practices in health communication campaigns (Aim 2). Recommendations and implications of our assessment are included in Chapter Four (Aim 3).

CHAPTER TWO

Rationale, Content, Design, and Dissemination of the Real Warriors Campaign

This chapter describes the rationale and theoretical basis for the RWC, followed by an overview of the activities undertaken by campaign staff to identify the target populations and to develop goals, messages, and materials. It concludes by providing a brief overview of campaign activities that support those goals, including the design of the campaign, development of campaign content, and dissemination and marketing of the campaign. The information in this chapter was derived from document review and discussions with RWC staff, as well as interviews with partner organizations.

Rationale for Developing the Real Warriors Campaign: Servicemembers Face Unique Barriers to Accessing Care for Mental Health Problems

Despite efforts from both the DoD and the Veterans Health Administration (VHA) to enhance mental health services, many servicemembers are still not regularly seeking needed care when they have mental health problems. Hoge et al. (2004) found that among soldiers and marines who met the screening criteria for a mental health problem, only 38 to 45 percent indicated an interest in receiving help and only 23 to 40 percent reported having received professional help in the past year. Similarly, Tanielian and Jaycox (2008) found that only 53 percent of servicemembers meeting the diagnostic criteria for PTSD or major depression had seen a physician or mental health provider.

Without appropriate treatment, these mental health problems can have wide-ranging and negative impacts on the quality of life and the social, emotional, and cognitive functioning of affected servicemembers. Such problems can also compound the costs of engaging in combat by increasing both medical costs for treating servicemembers who delay getting treatment and direct costs for replacing servicemembers who leave or are compelled to leave service before completing their contracts (Westphal, 2007). Servicemembers who suffer from PTSD or depression are more likely to have other mental health problems and to attempt suicide (Brady, Killeen, et al., 2000; Cavanagh, Carson, et al., 2003) and have higher rates of unhealthy behaviors including smoking, alcohol and drug use; overeating; and unsafe sex (Wulsin, Vaillant, et al., 1999; Breslau, Davis, et al., 2003; Grant, Stinson, et al., 2004; Schnurr, Hayes, et al., 2006; Feldner, Babson, et al., 2007). PTSD can negatively impact work performance and interpersonal relationships among servicemembers (Kessler, Walters, et al., 1998; Savoca and Rosenheck, 2000; Smith, Schnurr, et al., 2005). Veterans who suffer from major depression or PTSD have more difficulty securing and maintaining employment, which is a major component of successful reintegration into civilian life (Adler, Possemato, et al., 2011; Zivin, Bohnert, et al., 2011).

Two key barriers are frequently cited as keeping servicemembers from seeking care: concerns about the stigma associated with mental health problems and help-seeking, and fear of negative career repercussions (Greene-Shortridge, Britt, et al., 2007; Westphal, 2007). Hoge et al. (2004) found that servicemembers who screened positive for a mental health problem were twice as likely as those who screened negative to report concern about being stigmatized and about the barriers to accessing and receiving mental health services. There are also individual characteristics that have been shown to influence help-seeking behavior, including sex, age, and perceptions about the effectiveness of mental health treatment and perceived need for treatment (Vogt, 2011). Extended waiting times for appointments, lengthy paperwork, and difficulty navigating the health care system have all been found to reduce the likelihood that servicemembers will seek needed care (Dickstein, Vogt, et al., 2010; Vogt, 2011).

Research suggests that it is critical to look both at individual characteristics that predict help-seeking and at barriers within the system of care in order to reduce such barriers for servicemembers (Britt, Greene-Shortridge, et al., 2008). Once in the system of care, servicemembers might also have a bad experience with mental health providers or could receive inadequate treatment. One recent study of female veterans of OEF/OIF found that prior bad experiences with mental health providers was one of the most commonly cited barriers to care (Owens, Herrera, et al., 2009). Tanielian and Jaycox (2008) looked further at the treatment delivered to recently deployed servicemembers with mental health problems and found that just over half of servicemembers who sought care received minimally adequate treatment for their mental health disorder.

A review by Dickstein et al. of intervention strategies that address these barriers to care for servicemembers who have deployed suggested that the military should focus on five target areas to improve care-seeking behavior: "perceptions that care utilization is a sign of weakness; stereotypes about mental illness and mental health diagnoses (e.g., indicative of incompetence, dangerousness, or 'craziness'); self-blame (e.g., feeling responsible for having a mental illness); uncertainty about the signs and symptoms of mental illness; and uncertainty about the nature of treatment" (Dickstein, Vogt, et al., 2010, p. 231). Other research has underscored the influence that leaders have on servicemembers, suggesting that engaging leaders is a key strategy to improve help-seeking behaviors (Britt, Davison, et al., 2004).

Need for a Media Campaign to Encourage Servicemembers to Seek Care

The RWC was developed in response to Recommendation 5.1.1.1 of the 2007 Department of Defense Mental Health Task Force report (Defense Health Board Task Force on Mental Health, 2007), which stated: "The Department of Defense should implement an anti-stigma public education campaign, using evidence based techniques to provide factual information about mental disorders." A related recommendation in Section 5.1.3 of that report provides further impetus for the creation of the RWC, focusing on a need to embed training about mental health and psychological well-being throughout military life. This includes training military leaders, family members, and medical personnel. "Leaders, front-line supervisors, peers, friends, family members, health care providers and other helping agency members must all collaborate in building resilience, recognizing signs of distress and illness, serving as links to helping resources, and following up with those who have accepted or rejected assistance."

In response to the MHTF recommendations, DCoE held two summits with mental health leaders and servicemembers to identify priorities and the potential scope of a campaign and to help guide the development of a request for proposals to develop and manage the RWC. In 2008, DCoE released the request for proposals and the contract was subsequently awarded to Booz Allen Hamilton. Initial program development included a review of existing literature and public education campaigns, 14 focus groups with servicemembers representing different segments of the population (e.g., officers, female servicemembers, enlisted personnel), and consultation with experts to determine the most important areas of focus for the program. The final campaign was inspired by the National Institute of Mental Health's "Real Men, Real Depression" campaign, which focused on reducing stigma and assisting men in reaching out to access available mental health services (Rochlen, Whilde, et al., 2005). The Real Warriors Campaign was launched in May 2009.

Theoretical Basis of the Real Warriors Campaign

The RWC was based on the Health Belief Model (HBM) (see Figure 2.1). The HBM is a framework for motivating people to take positive health actions. It uses the desire to avoid a negative health consequence as a prime motivation and belief in positive outcomes as a reinforcing principle (Becker, 1974). It is built on four constructs: perceived susceptibility, perceived severity, perceived barriers, and perceived benefits.

Figure 2.1
Health Belief Model as Applied to the Real Warriors Campaign

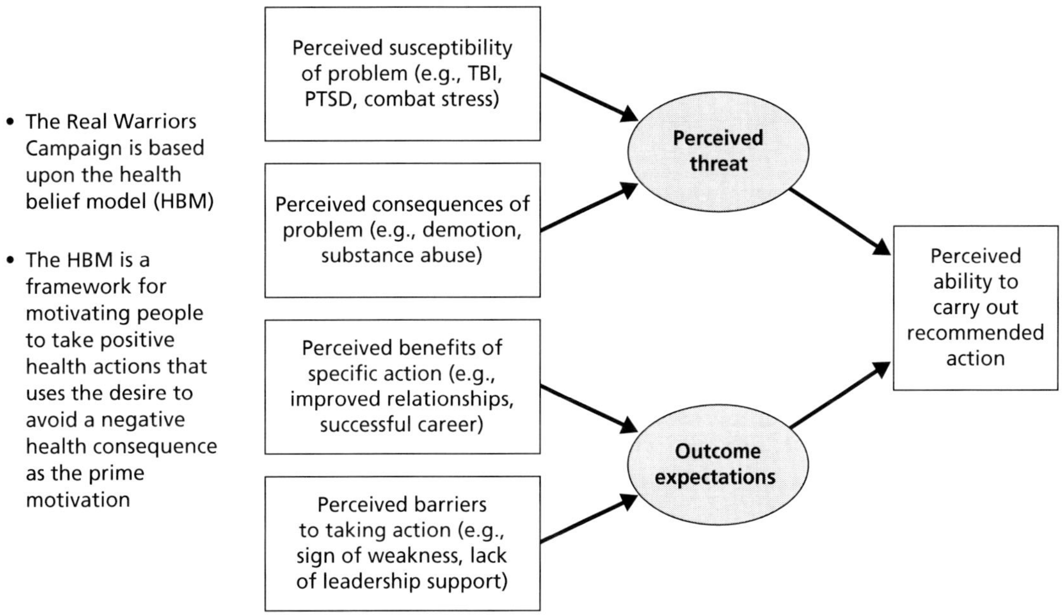

NOTE: This figure is modified from Becker's Health Belief Model (1974) and is reproduced with permission from the Real Warriors Campaign.
RAND *TR1176-2.1*

Design and Content of the Campaign: Target Populations, Campaign Goals, Messages, and Materials

Using the HBM as the campaign framework, RWC staff conducted literature reviews, focus groups, interviews, and market analysis to identify the threats perceived by servicemembers experiencing mental health concerns, the perceived and real motivators to taking action, the benefits and barriers to reaching out for care that exist within the military community, and tactics that would influence behavior change.

The literature review was used to identify key studies related to mental health in the military, mental health stigma, and help-seeking behavior (general help-seeking among males and help-seeking for mental health). RWC searched for peer-reviewed literature, DoD, Government Accountability Office, and Inspector General reports, and other task force reports (e.g., DoD Task Force on Mental Health) related to campaign target audiences. Staff used the following search terms: stigma, combat duty in Iraq and Afghanistan, barriers to care in the military community, mental health problems in OEF/OIF veterans, mental health in the military community, mental health in National Guard and Reserve, use of mental health services after combat, deployment stress, suicide prevention, stress in the military, peer to peer support programs, help-seeking among men, child and family, leaders' influence and attitudes, and public attitudes toward warrior care.

Additionally, RWC staff conducted a market analysis to identify existing mental health initiatives to ensure that the campaign would amplify and augment current efforts and avoid duplication. The market analysis included

- review and analysis of more than 50 programs, campaigns, and outreach efforts, both military and nonmilitary, that specifically target mental health issues
- development of an in-depth reference guide of the most significant health campaigns and a matrix of the tools and tactics used in each campaign, as well as the audiences targeted by each.

RWC staff also conducted eleven 90-minute focus groups made up of four to nine individuals each. Focus groups were held at key military and military health events, including the Association of Military Surgeons of the United States Annual Conference (November 2008), the Warrior Resilience Conference (November 2008), and the Suicide Prevention Conference (January 2009). Key informant interviews were conducted in September–December 2008 with 49 additional participants. Focus group and interview participants included representatives of the Army, Marine Corps, Navy, Air Force, Air National Guard, and Army National Guard in varying ranks, including both enlisted personnel and officers. Participants represented

- military mental health professionals who have provided care in a post-deployment setting
- previously deployed servicemembers who have sought treatment for PTSD or other mental health issues
- previously deployed servicemembers who have demonstrated a reluctance toward seeking treatment for PTSD and other mental health issues
- previously deployed line leaders from OEF/OIF
- previously deployed Reserve and Guard servicemembers from OEF/OIF

- spouses and other family members of servicemembers who have returned from deployment and exhibited PTSD symptoms.

All interviews and eight of the focus groups were conducted before any content for the RWC was designed. They focused on identifying perceived and/or real barriers to treatment, characterizing those who seek treatment and those reluctant to seek treatment, understanding the target audience for the campaign, and identifying types of messages and messengers that resonate with target audiences, and media for effectively delivering messages.

Three focus groups, held in January 2009, were used to test initial content, including imagery, messages, taglines, logos, and branding for the campaign. Participants were guided through discussions of the content to identify compelling content, discuss what they thought the content was trying to convey, and provide feedback on needed improvements to the content.

Information gathered from the literature review, focus groups, interviews, and market analysis was used to describe incidences of mental health concerns and potential differences among service branches and components, rates of perceived stigma and mental health service utilization, and fears about and perceived barriers to care. RWC staff used this information to inform campaign message development; to understand needs, differences, and communication preferences of target audiences; to identify tools and techniques for disseminating messages, including social marketing; and to aid in development of discussion guides for focus group and key informant interviews.

Target Populations

This research led to the identification of five relevant target populations for the campaign: active duty servicemembers, members of the Reserve or National Guard, veterans, families (including caregivers, adolescents, and children), and health professionals. The campaign serves all branches and components of the armed services. Although developed in response to concern regarding the mental health and psychological well-being of servicemembers returning from recent conflicts in Iraq and Afghanistan, the RWC is designed to serve any current or former military personnel and their family.

Campaign Goals

The RWC has four campaign goals that map to the four constructs in the HBM. The first goal of the campaign is to raise awareness about the signs and symptoms of mental health concerns. As a result, the RWC intends that knowledge about the prevalence of mental health problems among its target populations will improve their perceptions that they or someone they know could be susceptible to developing a mental health problem (perceived susceptibility). The second goal of the campaign is to raise awareness about the relative costs of inaction as compared with action in seeking help for mental health concerns. Improved awareness is intended to help the target populations accurately assess the consequences of seeking or not seeking help for a mental health problem (perceived consequences). The third goal is to raise expectations for positive outcomes for seeking support or treatment (perceived benefits). Finally, the campaign's fourth goal is to raise the target populations' awareness about the resources and services available for support and treatment, thereby lessening their perception of barriers to care (perceived barriers). Together, these four goals are designed to motivate servicemembers to seek appropriate help for mental health problems by lowering their perception of threat to seeking help and raising their perception of benefits.

Core Messages

The five core messages were designed to reinforce these goals by helping servicemembers, veterans, and their families understand that they are not alone in experiencing and dealing with mental health concerns and that effective resources for care and treatment are available and effective. These core messages are the following:

- Experiencing psychological stress as a result of deployment is common.
- Unlike visible wounds, psychological wounds and brain injuries are often invisible and can go untreated if not identified. Successful treatment and positive outcome are greatly assisted by early intervention.
- Servicemembers should know that they and their families should feel comfortable reaching out to their units and chain of command for support.
- Reaching out is a sign of strength that benefits servicemembers, their families, their units, and their services. Together, military leaders, servicemembers, families, and health professionals can spread the message that reaching out is a sign of strength.
- Warriors are not alone in coping with mental health concerns—there is a vast network of support and resources throughout each of the services, DoD, VA, and civilian communities. Help is available 24 hours a day, 7 days a week.

Campaign Activities and Materials

Messages, imagery, and resources are targeted to each service branch and each target audience (active duty servicemembers, members of the National Guard and Reserve, veterans, families, and health care providers) to demonstrate relevance to each specific audience and to provide targeted information and resources to each. For example, there are service-specific (i.e., using the same messaging, but different images for each service), posters and video profiles/PSAs, and audience-specific articles, materials, video profiles/PSAs, and resources displayed on the website.

Dissemination of the Real Warriors Campaign

The campaign reaches servicemembers, veterans, members of the National Guard and Reserve, families, and health care professionals through a variety of communication channels. These include the RWC website, social media, partnership activities, and conferences and events.

Website

The RWC website is the primary mode of disseminating information and materials. It features downloadable materials; e-cards or greeting cards that are sent via email; message boards where users can post questions and answer postings; video profiles of servicemembers who have sought help; PSAs; a live chat (available 24/7) with the DCoE Outreach Center; and more than 80 articles that provide specific tools, tips, and resources for the target populations. Each web page highlights contact information for the DCoE Outreach Center and the VA Veteran's Crisis Line. The campaign maintains a mobile version of the website for smartphone devices.

Partner Organizations

The RWC collaborates with a variety of DoD, service-branch, and federal organizations, as well as national and local not-for-profit organizations that share the campaign's mission and can help reach out to the target populations. Just over half of the partners are national-level organizations. Through regular communication and collaboration with these partners, the campaign seeks to increase its reach to target populations, gain credibility among partner members, offer the most relevant and up-to-date resources, and provide partners with campaign messages and easy, effective outreach mechanisms. As of July 2011, the campaign was connected with 153 partner organizations, and this number is steadily growing.

The campaign's partners include agencies and organizations that support the military community by providing information, resources, training, education, care, treatment, and/or advocacy for mental health problems. Each of these partners aligns with one or more of the campaign's goals, and each partner engages in one or more activities, including disseminating campaign information and materials, listing the campaign logo and/or web link on its website, and/or being listed by the RWC as a resource for information or services (e.g., employment, mental health, recreation; see Table 2.1).

The campaign approached approximately three-fourths of its partners to initiate a relationship, and the remaining partners approached the campaign. All partner relationships are based on a mutual agreement to work together. There is a formal application and evaluation process for new organizations, and approval of potential partners by DCoE leadership is

Table 2.1
Partner Organizations and Functions

	No. of Partner Organizations
Initiation	
Campaign initiated contact with partner	118
Partner initiated contact with campaign	35
Strategic Purpose(s) of Partnership with the RWC	
Create awareness about mental health concerns	127
Increase stakeholder knowledge of resources available	150
Facilitate access to care or remove barriers to care	133
Other, including involvement in campaign launch or serving as a local resource	35
Role(s) as Partner	
Lists the campaign logo and/or web link on its website	99
Publishes articles or news briefs about the campaign	33
Includes campaign updates in e-blasts, e-newsletters, social media and/or blogs	46
Disseminates or displays campaign materials (e.g., at events or in offices or clinics)	62
Is listed as a resource in the partner section of RWC website	153
Is listed as a resource in articles on the RWC website	52
Other, including conferences, roundtables, and briefings	15

required prior to developing a partner relationship. In early 2011, the RWC convened its first quarterly teleconference with partner organizations.

Conferences and Other Outreach Efforts

The campaign also disseminates information and materials to target populations through outreach efforts, including installation visits (e.g., during "game day" events), speaking engagements, and exhibitions at military and health industry related conferences and events (e.g., the Military Health System Conference and the American Psychiatric Association annual meeting). The campaign had an exhibition or presence at 32 conferences and events in 2009 and 41 in 2010.

CHAPTER THREE

Results of RAND's Assessment of the Real Warriors Campaign

This chapter presents results from our assessment of the RWC activities, addressing in particular the design, content, and dissemination of the campaign. We synthesize our findings from all six data sources, since multiple data sources contributed to our assessment in each content area. We also include a separate section on research and monitoring, given their critical implications for understanding the origins of the RWC as well as current and future revisions to the design of the campaign, content development, and dissemination strategies.

Although we synthesize findings across all data sources, the literature review primarily informed the dialogue and recommendations of the expert panel. The interviews with partner organizations were used to inform our assessment of the breadth of dissemination efforts and to elicit the recommendations from partner organizations. The content analysis was used primarily to assess the extent to which the design of the campaign is actually reflected in its content. The communication metrics were primarily used to assess the dissemination of the campaign. Document review and discussions with RWC staff were used to provide the description of the RWC on which this assessment is based. More information about each of these methods and the associated findings are contained in Appendixes B through F.

Campaign Design: Goals, Target Populations, and Messages of the Campaign

This section focuses on the foundation of the RWC, summarizing findings regarding the campaign's goals, target population, and core messages. Overall, the expert panel agreed that the RWC adheres to best practices in health communication campaigns, but had recommendations regarding how to strengthen the implementation and tailoring of campaign messages to better reach target populations.

Campaign Goals Are Clear, but They Are Not Clearly Stated in the Real Warriors Campaign Materials

Our review of the four campaign goals suggests that they are consistent with the Health Belief Model, which serves as the theoretical basis of the campaign. The goal of raising awareness about the signs and symptoms of mental health concerns, for example, helps to address perceived susceptibility. Raising awareness about the relative costs of inaction as compared with action helps to address perceived consequences of help-seeking. Raising expectations for positive outcomes helps to address the perceived benefits of help-seeking, and raising awareness about the resources and services available helps to address perceived barriers to seeking care.

When the goals of the campaign were provided to and discussed with the expert panel, the general sentiment was that these goals were appropriate and clear. However, members of the panel repeatedly noted that these goals are not stated on the RWC website or in the campaign materials. Because the goals are not clearly stated in campaign materials, partners of the RWC with whom we spoke had different perceptions of the purpose of the RWC. Some thought that it was to raise awareness of mental health issues and provide information for referrals; others viewed it as an anti-stigma campaign whose main goal was reducing stigma around help-seeking. Another explicitly noticed a shift in the campaign's goals since its inception—from targeting stigma to a much broader idea, making the current goals less clear. Other partners were unsure of the goals and objectives of the campaign.

> Is this a campaign, an informational website, a psychological referral service, a hotline? [Representative from a partner organization]

Expert panelists and RWC partners both recommended that the campaign goals be clearly stated on the homepage of the website and on relevant materials to help users better understand the purpose of the campaign and what it offers.

The goal that drew the most attention from both partners and expert panels was raising awareness about the resources and services that are available for support and treatment. A limited number of RWC partners questioned whether the campaign, as an information and referral source, is necessary or helpful given the large number of resources available and the lists that help identify such resources. The expert panel, however, felt that raising awareness of resources was an important goal but noted that its execution in the campaign materials could have been strengthened. Both partners and experts noted a missed opportunity for the RWC to take a more proactive approach to disseminating information. Although both partners and the expert panel felt that it was good to have a wide range of resources available, they noted that the breadth of information and resources on the website was overwhelming, potentially leaving the user unsure of a specific course of action. Little information, for example, was provided to help users understand which resource(s) would best meet their needs. The expert panel and partners noted that family members and health professionals in particular were given little guidance as to next steps for developing a plan of action.

While the RWC goals were well formulated, had a strong theoretical basis, and were considered to be appropriate and clear, RWC partners and expert panelists felt that the dissemination of those goals could be strengthened.

Health Professionals Are a Less Relevant Target Population

In general, the expert panel felt that the target audiences for the campaign were relevant, although some members felt that the goals of the campaign did not align as well with health professionals as with other target audiences. Health professionals, particularly those with expertise in mental health, are likely aware of the signs and symptoms of mental health concerns, the relative costs of inaction as opposed to action, and the benefits of seeking support or treatment. While health professionals may use the site to learn about available resources and support, much of the content in the health professionals section of the website is related to evidence-based practices, becoming a TRICARE provider, and understanding the military culture. While these issues are clearly important and related to the campaign, they fall outside the scope of the campaign's goals as currently stated. Campaign metrics also suggest that

> The Real Warriors Campaign provides resources and information to support quality mental health and healthcare for our nation's servicemembers. Reaching out for help is a sign of strength. We're here to help, and you are not alone. [Expert panel member.]

RWC partners and expert panelists also observed that the campaign's messaging was not equally compelling for all groups. Some felt that the messaging was not as compelling for family members, especially since they are likely to visit the RWC website to learn how to support a servicemember in their family, rather than to seek help themselves. One expert panel member also had a difficult time figuring out what the messages were for health professionals, further suggesting that this population—although clearly relevant to the issue of mental health—may be outside the scope of the campaign.

Other expert panelists with experience working with servicemembers in different branches of service felt that the campaign did a better job on messaging for active duty soldiers but that messaging for the National Guard and Reserve component and the other branches of service fell short.

> The messages are really not compelling for every branch except the Army. Anyone who felt like a marine or a Guard member would feel like "they haven't really identified what my issues are." [Expert panel member]

Although experts did feel, overall, that the core messages of the campaign were relevant and clear as developed, the challenge was in the execution and tailoring of those messages to resonate with and be actionable for each of the target populations and subpopulations within those groups.

Campaign Content

This section describes our findings about the content of the RWC website and materials and summarizes partner and expert panelist feedback about the extent to which the RWC's content is adequate across target populations and effective in achieving RWC goals.

Video Profiles Are the Most Compelling Content

Both experts and partners felt strongly that the video profiles containing personal stories of servicemembers struggling with mental health problems were the "heart" of the campaign. Both groups consistently described these profiles as "compelling." The videos were widely considered the most useful campaign tool for delivering its messages. Communication metrics indicate that users spend the most time on the multimedia pages of the website (an average of 35 seconds as compared with an average of 13 seconds on other RWC pages), further supporting these sentiments. Our content analysis of the RWC website found that the video profiles were the only materials that communicated the RWC's messages about the cost of action versus inaction, further underscoring their importance.

Partners also reported receiving positive feedback directly from their constituents on the videos. In order to better showcase the videos, partners and expert panelists suggested moving these to the homepage of the website and using streaming video to run a continuous loop showing the video content. Partners suggested some improvements to the videos, such as including more veterans from earlier generations and previous wars to serve as examples of success stories, and a greater inclusion of women and junior enlisted servicemembers.

Since the data collection period for this study ended, the RWC website has been updated to position the videos more centrally on the website.

The Breadth of the Content Dilutes the Campaign's Key Messages

Partners and expert panelists indicated that there was too much content on the website, describing it as "overly dense" and causing "information overload," and remarked that the long lists of links, resources, and materials did not provide enough direction to users on how to prioritize the information. Experts remarked that the lists were not categorized and that there was no hierarchy to the lists, making it difficult for users to differentiate between items on the lists.

> I think the key question is "Is more information better?" And what we're saying is no. [Expert panel member]

> They just put together a hodgepodge of stuff. It's too broad, too watered down, and too murky. [Expert panel member]

> They tried to do everything, instead of focusing on the key messages. Here's everything we know! . . . they sort of lost that focus. [Expert panel member]

The breadth of information and resources on the website were described as overwhelming for users, and the expert panel suggested that users may leave the website being unsure about a specific course of action. Even with the significant breadth of materials, experts indicated that while the RWC website and materials clearly conveyed to servicemembers that they should reach out if they need help, it stopped short of providing specific courses of action other than contacting the DCoE Outreach Center or the VA Veteran's Crisis Line. Panelists noted that providing a breadth of informational resources may not translate to increasing help-seeking behaviors.

> I don't think you can confuse providing a list of resources with conveying a solution or a clear course of action. A list of resources the warrior may tend to skim, but what I was hoping for was something more than "pick one of these and go for it" but more "here's what you do next." I didn't think a list of resources was enough to carry the day. [Expert panel member]

> If the solution is "reach out, seek help" then yes, that was very clear to me. A more concrete course of action was not. Talk to your commander, or you can reach your unit counselor in this way, oftentimes those more concrete courses of action have been shown to increase people's likelihood of actually doing that [engaging in the recommended behavior]. [Expert panel member]

Expert panelists noted that family members, in particular, were not provided with clear courses of action.

The Depth of Content Is Uneven Across Goals and Target Populations

Our content analysis found that the materials on the RWC website primarily supported two goals: (1) raising awareness of mental health services and (2) raising awareness of other resources. The extent to which the RWC raised expectations of positive outcomes, however, varied by target population. For example, there were no materials directed toward Reserve and Guard servicemembers to raise expectations of positive outcomes; however, materials with this purpose were included in the active duty and veterans pages. As previously mentioned, the video profiles were the only materials on the RWC website that communicated messages concerning the costs of inaction as opposed to action.

Much of the website content was not directly relevant to any of the campaign goals. Our content analysis of website articles directed at each target population found that between 34 percent and 73.6 percent of the articles directed at specific target populations did not explicitly support campaign goals (34 percent of the articles for active duty were not relevant; 56 percent for veterans; 62 percent for Guard and Reserve; 71 percent among health professionals; and 74 percent for families). Many of the most frequently viewed articles were also not relevant to the goals of the RWC. For example, several of the most frequently viewed materials in 2010 described how to apply for a discharge upgrade, provided details on April as the "month of the military child," and talked about how to prepare children for deployment. While all of these are important topics for servicemembers and their families, they are not directly relevant to the goals of the campaign.

Coverage across target populations was also uneven, with more of the website and materials focusing on the active duty population. The majority of the multimedia tools were designed for the active duty population (41 out of the 49 items), with no videos and only two brochures relevant for health professionals. Articles were also more heavily weighted toward active duty (n=26), as compared with Reserve and Guard (n=13), veterans (n=16), families (n=19), or health professionals (n=7).

In particular, the expert panel felt that the lack of emphasis that the RWC placed on the Reserve and Guard population was a missed opportunity.

> The National Guard and Reserve page could be more immediate and relevant—saying they "have unique challenges balancing their military service with civilian life" [as stated on the website] is stating the obvious. There's got to be a more compelling way to package this information. Well, quite honestly, what I would do is pull Guard/Reserve out entirely and give them their own site. One of the biggest problems is to put all these groups together—It's just not doing them justice. [Representative from a partner organization]

The expert panelists noted that there are few other campaigns that target the Guard and Reserve populations and felt that the RWC could be a valuable resource. Communication metrics suggest that the number of page views for Guard and Reserve materials is growing at a much slower pace than materials for the other target populations (see Figure 3.1).

Updated Content Is Essential

Some of the expert panelists expressed concern that the content of the website was quickly becoming outdated. Several of the links to resources and other materials were no longer active or working. The panel suggested that rather than try to continually update the videos or maintain an extensive site with many links to external partners that can quickly become outdated, the RWC could link to fewer but more strategic connections that will remain current or that regularly update their material.

> Don't build something that's going to get out of date; you can't afford to do that. [Servicemembers] are too aware that the war changes every year. [Expert panel member]

The expert panel also emphasized that the RWC should determine whether the website intends to have users return regularly or to serve as a first stop to funnel new users to other resources. If the website is intended to have regular users, the RWC may want to update the website more regularly so that users are interacting with dynamic content. However, if the website is primarily designed to funnel new users to other resources, it would be preferable for the website to remain static and be more clearly tailored to new users' potential interests. Several panelists indicated that the website could potentially serve both purposes by having a single specific location on the website where a limited amount of information is continually updated for regular users.

Campaign Dissemination

This section focuses on the RWC's dissemination of messages and materials through its various communication channels. These include the campaign website, social media, partnership activities, and conferences and events. As noted above, the RWC website was redesigned after we conducted partner discussions. We have noted areas where this redesign may impact our findings.

The Real Warriors Campaign Website Is Useful, but Navigation Is a Challenge for Some

Several partner organizations provided positive feedback about the look and feel of the website and perceived it to be a useful means for widely disseminating information and materials. However, partners provided mixed feedback about website navigability. Although a small number of partners found the website easy to navigate or had received such feedback from their constituents, a majority of partners commenting on navigability reported experiencing difficulties while perusing the website. One partner reported that their constituents were unable to find the information they needed, even when it was available on the RWC website. As this partner noted,

> It was very hard to navigate the website. I've had a couple constituents ask me something related to the campaign . . . usually very general inquiries. And I had to go to the campaign [staff] directly to find out. The campaign in turn has said those things are on the website, and indeed they were. [Representative from a partner organization]

To improve navigability of the website, experts suggested that a statement on the home page describing how to navigate the website would help guide users. In addition, experts suggested that adding a rotating carousel outlining the website's offerings, creating a "crawler" on the home page with key messages and components, and adding a resources library would help to maximize the delivery of existing content.

Some partners and panelists also expressed concern that the website may be too passive a channel for effective dissemination of information. Panelists, for example, suggested that the campaign consider using technologies that actively respond to viewers' actions or "build relationships" with return visitors as an avenue for increasing user interactivity. As one expert suggested,

> There's a technology that Amazon.com uses—smart technology—if people are looking at different things, the site could say hey, I see you're interested in this. [Expert panel member]

While the RWC website is a potentially helpful tool for reaching the campaign's target audiences, panelists felt that key components of the site should be better highlighted and suggested technological solutions to increase website navigability and interactivity.

Social Media Channels Are Not Fully Utilized

The campaign disseminates information through a number of social media channels, including Facebook, Twitter, YouTube, and online message boards. Facebook and Twitter are used to disseminate messages and materials to military personnel and their families. Messages and materials include advice on reintegration after deployment, support forums, and a variety of resources targeted toward users who subscribe or opt to receive updates from the campaign. In addition, the campaign's Facebook page and Twitter feed offer interactive discussion tools through which users can post information and comments directly to the campaign pages and interact with the campaign staff and other subscribers. YouTube features a promotional channel through which video PSAs are posted online to direct viewers to the campaign website. The campaign also hosts its own discussion forum through online message boards on the campaign website. These message boards allow website visitors and members to post questions to the military community and interact with a network of military personnel, families, and professional care staff.

A few partners provided positive feedback about these social networking activities. Some stated that their constituents had conveyed positive feedback about these communication channels. Other partners expressed satisfaction with the campaign's social media activities based on their own engagement (e.g., direct partner interaction with the campaign through Facebook).

A few partners suggested that social media should be utilized more by the campaign, and the campaign's communication metrics support this recommendation. The campaign's number of Facebook fans includes a slowly increasing population of just over 3,000—a small number in relation to the multitude of individuals composing the campaign's five target populations. The number of campaign Twitter followers is increasing, with RWC tweets remaining consistent and re-tweets increasing. We were unable to discern the cause of the increase in re-tweets. This may be an area for RWC to examine further to determine if tweet increases were related to changes in the type or format of campaign materials. YouTube views are also increasing steadily over time. Message boards, however, have exhibited a decline in the number of new posts and new topics.

Although most of the campaign's social media tools are viewed as useful by its partners and are growing in popularity among target audiences, utilization is still limited, and some of these channels appear to be more useful than others.

Not All Partners Are Actively Engaged

Communication metrics suggest that the roles of partners vary significantly. Fifty-nine percent of all partners are *actively* engaged in disseminating campaign information materials and resources through articles, news briefs, e-blasts, e-newsletters, social media, or blogs, or at venues such as conferences, events, offices or clinics (see Table 2.1).

While 45 percent of partners list the campaign logo and/or web link on their websites, only 7 percent have that link on their homepage. Of the 26 partners with whom we held discussions, three felt that they did not know enough about the campaign or have enough interaction with the campaign to provide input.

Partner Organizations Want More Interaction with the Campaign

Approximately two-thirds of the partners we spoke with made suggestions for improvement of the campaign's partnership program. Many partners expressed a desire to strengthen their relationship with the campaign. Some partners, for example, had seldom interacted with the campaign and were unsure of the expectations of their organization as a campaign partner.

> [RWC] needs to tell me who they are and where my relationship with them is supposed to be. [Representative from a partner organization]

Other partners felt that their relationship with the campaign was "there in name" but did not have much depth to it.

> There's a lot of talk about partnering, but there's no real partnering . . . no partnering with teeth in it. [Representative from a partner organization]

> I sign up and I'm a partner. I have their logo on our website, and I get their newsletter, but in terms of involvement, I don't know what that would look like. [Representative from a partner organization]

Likewise, many partners thought the campaign should deepen rather than broaden its partnerships.

> What they actually need is meaningful partnerships. Just because you have 300 people on your list doesn't mean you've got meaningful partnerships. [Representative from a partner organization]

Several partners viewed their lack of interaction with the campaign as a missed opportunity to share information and learn more about how the campaign operates and is structured. For example, some partners were not aware that they could order/receive materials from the campaign. Instead, they thought they had to download and print materials themselves and reported not having the money to do so. Other partners lacked a clear sense of distinction between the RWC and DCoE. When asked about the RWC, these partners frequently provided responses pertaining to DCoE rather than the campaign itself. One partner thought that a primary purpose of the campaign was to promote DCoE's achievements.

Several partners suggested that the campaign get to know its partner organizations and the services they offer in order to better leverage their skills and resources. They also noted that if the RWC were aware of its partners' services and resources, it could then connect users who are in need of services to specific organizations or provide recommendations better tailored to users' geographic locations and needs. Currently, the RWC website does not differentiate partner organizations by the different populations or geographic regions they serve. Therefore, a user from Philadelphia, for example, could try to access resources from a partner organization that only services residents of California. This situation, reported by at least one partner organization as actually occurring, could discourage servicemembers from seeking additional services, ultimately working counter to the goals of the RWC.

Many partners felt that their relationships with the campaign have not been mutually supportive. Some stated that they support the campaign but that the campaign has not provided them with significant support. Others perceived the campaign to be unfamiliar with their organization's activities or felt that "no one is listening to ideas from the field." Most often, these partners' sentiments were not that the RWC staff is unwilling to listen and assist but that little structure is in place enabling the campaign to do so. A few partners suggested that the campaign reach out to its partners to learn about their concerns and priorities. Early in 2011, the campaign held the first of what are intended to be regular conference calls with partners. While some of the partners reported participating in the first call, others were unaware that it had occurred.

> I don't think they've gathered the partners together, hosted a day retreat to find out what partners think of the campaign. [Representative from a partner organization]

Partners who did participate in the conference call found it to be helpful in creating dialogue and information exchange between partners and the campaign.

Partner Organizations Want More Interaction with Other Partners

Several partners felt that their relationships with other partnering organizations could be strengthened. They noted that they have had limited interaction with other partners and viewed this as a missed opportunity to share information or collaborate.

> There may be some very natural ways that we could put ourselves together as program partners if we all sat down in [the] same place at [the] same time and are told to brainstorm . . . but we are all locked in our own disparate worlds wishing we could do more. [Representative from a partner organization]

Some partners indicated that they would like to see partner organizations "clustered" in smaller groups based on geographic region or target population and to have a point of contact from the RWC assigned to each region. They felt that this would foster more productive and effective interaction among partners—in particular, allowing for more face-to-face interaction.

While campaign partners occupy a critical role in the dissemination of information and materials, these partners are not fully utilized and engaged to the extent possible. Partners would like the campaign to provide them with more information and updates, to better highlight them and the services they provide, and to foster partner-to-partner collaboration.

Conferences and Events Are Useful for Dissemination, but Could Be Improved

Some partners expressed positive feedback about the RWC's activities at conferences and events.

> [RWC staff] spoke at our . . . conference [and] showed how the campaign helps; [they] used videos and PSAs, and we had a very positive response. [Representative from a partner organization]

Others indicated that the campaign could benefit from a general increase in face-to-face outreach with its target populations.

> [RWC] need[s] to send out inspirational speakers as a way to put a face to the campaign. [Representative from a partner organization]

> For the outreach portion there is no substitute for shoe leather. [Representative from a partner organization]

> There's got to be an interpersonal basis. [Representative from a partner organization]

Partners also suggested that the campaign increase its presence at conferences or events to establish a "presence more as a leader." Some recommended that the RWC host its own seminar or conference.

> [RWC] need[s] to get out there in front—as it is its own unique thing—rather than attending these other conferences. [Representative from a partner organization]

Communication metrics also suggest that the campaign may be able to improve its dissemination of information and materials at conferences. On average, few conference attendees visit an RWC booth if it is not tied to a DCoE display. While 21.2 percent of conference attendees visit a conference booth if there is only a DCoE presence, only 2.2 percent visit the booth if the RWC is there without DCoE presence. Approximately 7 percent visit the booth if both RWC and DCoE are represented. However, material distribution and listserv sign-up is highest when visitors come to a booth that clearly states the RWC name. Approximately 20 percent of conference attendees who visit an RWC booth sign up to be on the listserv. Approximately 10–15 percent sign up if the booth has a DCoE presence as well. In addition, communication metrics show that the average number of educational and promotional materials disseminated is over 800 per event for RWC-only booths and 140 pieces of material for DCoE-only booths.

While the campaign's current efforts to disseminate information and materials at conferences, events, and other face-to-face venues appear to be useful and well received, partner feedback and communication metrics suggest that there is room for improvement to the strategies used and that additional venues should be considered.

Research and Ongoing Monitoring

This section describes our findings of how the RWC has used research and monitoring to better target efforts and to improve and refine ongoing efforts.

Research Should Continue to Be Utilized to Build Campaign Goals and Messages

As described in Chapter Two, RWC staff reported using both research and stakeholder analysis as the basis for developing campaign messages and tactics. Research activities included a literature review of at least 15 key studies related to mental health issues in the military, and a review of at least 50 military and nonmilitary programs and outreach efforts that address mental health, including post-traumatic stress disorder.

RWC staff also conducted 11 focus group sessions and 49 key informant interviews with military mental health professionals who have provided care in a postdeployment setting; previously deployed active duty, Reserve and Guard servicemembers and line leaders from OEF/OIF; and spouses and other family members of servicemembers who have returned from deployment and exhibited PTSD symptoms. These research activities were conducted during the fall of 2008 and winter of 2009.

As a result of this research the RWC staff decided to do the following:

- Create video profiles of servicemembers and veterans from a variety of ranks and branches of service who have sought treatment or reached out for support and who continue to have successful military or civilian careers. The formative research suggested that servicemembers wanted real-world examples of other servicemembers who were able to have a successful career after receiving treatment for a mental health problem.
- Tailor messages, imagery, and resources to each branch of service and target audience. For example, there are service-specific posters, video profiles, PSAs, eCards, and resources; and audience-specific web articles, materials, video profiles, PSAs, and resources. Focus group findings suggested that, to be fully engaged, target populations would need to "see individuals like themselves" in the RWC messages, imagery, and resources.
- Post the RWC website on a civilian URL (.net), rather than a .mil or .gov website. Focus group findings suggested that servicemembers were reluctant to visit DoD websites for information on mental health because of concerns that these websites were under surveillance.

Communication Metrics Are Not Fully Leveraged

The RWC currently collects and reports a range of communication metrics, including metrics that reflect how widely materials are being disseminated (e.g., media and print mentions of the campaign), utilization of the website (e.g., number of hits), and outreach by campaign staff (e.g., newsletter, social media). A full list of these metrics is included in Appendix E.

Although these metrics were being collected, the RWC was not using the information from those metrics to help guide strategic decisions about the campaign. As of August 2011, the RWC had only utilized communication metrics to report to DCoE about the progress of the campaign and was in the process of hiring a consultant to help analyze and more fully utilize these metrics.

RWC staff report utilizing current communication metrics to determine whether the campaign is meeting its objectives and to inform future campaign materials, developments, and initiatives. Although current communication metrics show how many people were reached, there is no information about what proportion of the target population this number represents.

Mechanisms to Gather Regular Feedback Are Lacking, and More Usability Testing Is Needed

Both partners and expert panelists suggested that the RWC needs to regularly seek feedback on its website and materials and on the relevance of the messages it disseminates. Many partners felt that while the RWC was doing a good job of pushing information out, it lacked feedback mechanisms to determine whether the materials were well received or successful in supporting the campaign's goals. The expert panel suggested that the RWC could include a pop-up survey for website users as one way to gather feedback. One partner suggested that the RWC could solicit feedback from partners via its newsletter or monthly teleconference.

In 2009, the RWC reported conducting a heuristic evaluation and focus groups with members of the Army, Navy, and Marine Corps to assess whether the website mock-up designs complied with recognized usability principles or heuristics (Nielsen, 1994). Other than this assessment, which was conducted before the campaign launched, the RWC has not conducted any usability testing of the website (personal communication from the RWC staff to the lead author, September 27, 2011). However, the RWC did report incorporating changes to improve the usability of the website based on feedback from our partners as well as webmaster email feedback (for example, RWC staff changed "Multimedia" as a menu option to "Videos" based on feedback). Our expert panel also suggested that a thorough usability test would help the RWC identify areas for website improvement. Panelists stressed the importance of usability testing of a website at several key points in time, including before a website is launched, before any redevelopment efforts, repeatedly while a website is active (particularly as new content is incorporated into an existing website), and when analysis of communication metrics shows a slow-down in website traffic. Usability testing can help assess how users interact with the website and identify areas where users get lost or have difficulty finding what they are looking for. Regular usability testing could help the RWC validate findings, described above, that specifically suggest that the RWC website is difficult to navigate because it contains too much information.

Beyond the communication metrics, described above, the RWC does not collect any ongoing process or outcome evaluation. Evaluation is critical to assessing whether the campaign is achieving its goals and having a measurable impact on servicemembers and their families.

Limitations of Our Assessment

Our evaluation was limited in scope to an assessment of campaign activities. We focused our efforts on the core elements of the campaign—its goals, target populations, and core messages; the ways in which those elements were executed to create meaningful, relevant, and actionable campaign materials; and the methods and strategies used by the campaign to disseminate those messages. While this approach provided important insights into the strengths and opportunities for improvement of campaign activities specifically, it does not provide information on the effectiveness of the campaign in achieving short-term or intermediate outcomes, such as gains in knowledge or changes in perceptions related to help-seeking. Further, our assessment does not provide information about whether individuals decided to seek help for mental health concerns as a result of the campaign's efforts. While answering those questions is important and should be undertaken in the future, this study was designed as a preliminary assessment because the campaign itself is fairly new. Further, at the time our assessment was conducted, the contract to manage the campaign was being re-competed, suggesting that additional evaluation activities would be valuable after management changes and any content or dissemination redesign take place.

Another limitation of our evaluation is that we were not able to collect data from target audiences due to time, budgetary, and logistical constraints. Although many of our findings were related to the tone of messages and whether those messages were relevant and compelling, we did not verify those findings with members of the target audiences. The RWC partners and expert panelists, however, do have a long history of working with and serving servicemembers and their families or have expertise in media campaigns.

A final implication of not collecting data from target audiences is that it limited our ability to answer questions about the campaign's penetration rates. Although the RWC does collect a range of metrics to provide a sense of the potential reach of the campaign through various dissemination channels, this is not the same as conducting a systematic assessment of the campaign's penetration rate or the level of exposure of servicemembers to the campaign. Assessing penetration rates would require a large-scale survey of a representative sample of the target populations of the RWC.

CHAPTER FOUR

Recommendations to Improve Future Design and Dissemination of the Real Warriors Campaign

This chapter summarizes our recommendations for improving the RWC. It is organized into sections that focus on (1) the design and content of the campaign, (2) dissemination efforts, and (3) recommendations for improving the RWC's use of research and evaluation. In each section, we begin with those recommendations that are relatively easier to implement, followed by those that will take greater effort and should be considered as part of a long-term improvement strategy or during any significant redevelopment efforts. We recognize that the RWC may not be able to implement all of these recommendations, but we offer them as ideas for consideration as the RWC is being continually improved and refined. It is also possible that the awareness of an external evaluation and the process of re-competing the RWC contract in the fall of 2011 may have already prompted some changes in the campaign between the time of our assessment and publication of this report. As a result, some of the recommendations may have been addressed. Therefore, our recommendations should be considered in light of any recent changes to the campaign.

Recommendations to Improve Design and Content of the Real Warriors Campaign

We recommend the following changes to the RWC design and content that, based on our assessment, could improve the effectiveness of the RWC.

Recommendation 1.1. Clearly state the goals and core messages of the Real Warriors Campaign on the website. This is a relatively easy and inexpensive recommendation to implement, but it could help to greatly improve users' understanding of the purpose and intent of the campaign.

Recommendation 1.2. Review content and links to ensure that they are still current. RWC staff should systematically review the website content on a regular basis to identify inactive links. For example, setting a schedule to regularly click through all the links listed on each resource page would help identify resource links that have become inactive. This review could be part of the regular usability testing described in more detail under recommendation 3.2. Servicemembers should be engaged to help RWC identify content that is outdated.

Recommendation 1.3. Streamline existing content to ensure it aligns with goals and key messages. The RWC should make an effort to streamline the content on its website to primarily include materials that help to further campaign goals or messages. Our content analysis found that only the materials directed toward active duty servicemembers fully addressed the campaign goals and messages. Ongoing monitoring of the alignment between campaign goals, messages, and materials is critical to ensure that the website retains its focus. This could include instituting a review process by which new materials are thoroughly vetted for alignment with a particular campaign, goal, message, and target population.

Recommendation 1.4. Base the development of new goals and messages on findings from objective data sources, such as the Mental Health Advisory Team (MHAT) biannual survey. As the needs of the military shift over time, the RWC will need to adapt its goals to meet these needs. Future changes to campaign goals should be based on identified changes in the needs of the target audiences. For example, as servicemembers' awareness of the availability of mental services increases, the RWC may wish to lessen efforts focused on raising this awareness. Data from objective sources, such as the MHAT, should be used to ensure that changes to the RWC are made specifically in response to needs of the target populations.

Recommendation 1.5. Optimize the web layout of existing content. The RWC should revisit its website design to enhance navigation and to highlight the video profiles. Our expert panelists offered several suggestions along these lines, including adding a statement on the homepage describing how to navigate the website, adding a rotating carousel outlining the website's offerings, creating a "crawler" on the home page with key messages and components, and adding a resources library. The expert panel discussed The Courage to Care, Courage to Talk website (www.couragetotalk.org), which has a streaming video on the homepage that the panelists found to be a compelling layout.

Recommendation 1.6. Improve the tailoring of website content to specific target populations. The website content needs to resonate with target populations, and needs to be organized so that target populations can find materials they are looking for. Ensuring that the RWC recognizes differences not only between its target populations but also among servicemembers who differ in age, gender, or culture is critical to the campaign's success. Opportunities for improvement include creating an improved home page that helps direct users to the information they are seeking. Healthfinder.gov is a good example of an existing portal that uses this approach. Also, the RWC may wish to consider using smart technology that helps direct users, based on their current page, to other pages that are likely to be of interest to them. This provides the opportunity to introduce users to new materials that they might not have been thinking about or known they would benefit from. In tailoring website content, the RWC may wish to revisit whether health professionals are a viable target population for the campaign and potentially remove them from the campaign's efforts.

Recommendations to Improve the Dissemination of the Real Warriors Campaign

Several recommendations for how the RWC can improve the reach and effectiveness of its dissemination emerged from our findings.

Recommendation 2.1. Enhance and grow the social media channels that are most effective. Social media are gaining in popularity as fast and relatively inexpensive means to reach broad audiences. The RWC collects campaign metrics that help it look at people's use of social media. These metrics should be regularly monitored to identify and bolster the social media efforts that are effective. For example, the RWC could review the content of re-tweets and Facebook posting to determine what materials from the RWC website are most frequently being commented on. These materials could tell the RWC something about the individuals using their social media channels. The RWC also could augment its existing social media metrics by regularly collecting information about which populations (e.g., age, gender, membership in a target group) are the highest users of social media and are more likely to respond to given social media. This information could be used by the RWC to tailor its social media efforts to maximize the impact of its dissemination efforts.

Recommendation 2.2. Become more proactive in the dissemination of information. Partners and expert panelists felt that the RWC could greatly increase its visibility by being more proactive. Hosting a conference or a seminar at an ongoing conference, engaging in outreach efforts, and proactively synthesizing and disseminating relevant information to partners could all help the RWC be seen as more of a leader in this content area. Partners also consistently emphasized the importance of face-to-face contact with the campaign to promote relationship building among partnering organizations.

Recommendation 2.3. Utilize partners more effectively. Partners and panelists offered several suggestions for how the RWC could better leverage existing partnerships:

- More interaction between the RWC and partner organizations. This could include highlighting partners more prominently in RWC newsletters or on the website and regularly keeping partners up-to-date on the campaign.
- Segment or cluster partner organizations by geographic region, target population, or type of services offered. Ensure that these groups foster interaction among partners as well as with the campaign. The RWC should continue to hold quarterly conference calls and may want to consider having additional calls for each cluster of organizations.
- Make the availability of free print materials more visible to partners. Some partners were not aware that they could order or receive materials from the campaign. Instead, they thought they needed to download and print materials themselves and reported not having the money to do so.
- Increase the number of partner organizations that link to the RWC, and improve the placement of the RWC link on partner organization websites. Some partners placed the RWC link prominently on their homepage; others had it listed on pages that required several clicks to access.

If the RWC is concerned about staff having limited time to engage more deeply with existing partners, the campaign could implement a tiered partnership model. In a tiered model, there could be a small group of partners that are most critical to the campaign mission. RWC staff could regularly engage these partners by having face-to-face meetings at least annually to strategically reach out to target populations. The next tier could include organizations outside the mental health or social service system (e.g., recreational organizations) that servicemembers regularly access. The RWC could target educational materials toward the staff of these organizations and could request that these organizations run banner ads for the RWC on their websites. The final tier could include partner organizations that the RWC engages in a more limited fashion, primarily with cross-listed weblinks and logos or with dissemination of campaign materials on a more ad hoc basis.

Recommendations to Improve the Real Warriors Campaign's Use of Research and Evaluation

To improve the RWC's ability to conduct continuous quality improvement, monitor progress, and assess its short- and long-term impacts, we recommend the following actions.

Recommendation 3.1. Solicit regular feedback from partners. Our partner discussions revealed that partners were interested in providing feedback to the RWC, but did not feel comfortable proactively contacting the campaign to provide feedback. We suggest that the RWC consider collecting data from partners on a more regular basis. For example, the RWC could send an email survey to partner organizations every six months to get their feedback.

Recommendation 3.2. Engage in regular usability testing of the website. Although the RWC conducted research to help build campaign goals and messages, there has been limited usability testing of the website post launch. Regular usability testing should be conducted, particularly as content is updated.

Recommendation 3.3. Convene an ongoing expert or advisory panel to help the campaign stay current and highlight key issues. The expert panelists expressed interest in continuing to participate in an ongoing advisory panel to help the RWC make strategic decisions about how to improve, refine, and enhance the website and materials. The RWC could also consider convening a panel composed of target audience members to be involved in regular assessment of content and usability testing of the website.

Recommendation 3.4. Use improved communication metrics to conduct ongoing monitoring. Standard metrics regularly collected by the RWC provide counts of website users and social media exposure, but do not provide RWC staff with a true indicator of what proportion of the target audience is being reached or the impact of the RWC on target audiences. Although there are no gold standard communication metrics, we recommend that the RWC assess the feasibility of substituting or enhancing existing communication metrics to include the following types of metrics:

- **Nielsen online campaign ratings.** Nielsen has developed a new approach to assess online content that produces reach, frequency, and gross rating points statistics. Because the Nielsen online ratings were developed in September 2010, their validity and utility is not yet established. But they may provide better information to the RWC than has previously been available about the proportion of their target audience reached, information the RWC was not collecting as of October 2011.
- **Social media mentions of the RWC.** The RWC should also consider communication metrics that assess if the RWC is mentioned in online interactions (e.g., in blogs, Facebook pages, Tweets) outside of the RWC's own website—these social media mentions, also known as "chatter" or "buzz," are an indicator not only of the reach of the RWC, but of its population engagement with target audiences. Assessing the number of times a product, advertising campaign, television show, etc. is mentioned in social media is rapidly emerging as a method that complements and expands upon the information provided by standard campaign ratings (Dumenco, 2011). This technique of assessing whether a specific product is mentioned by Facebook users' regular postings or other online venues is widely utilized by public health communication campaigns to help determine their reach (Andreasen, 1994).

Recommendation 3.5. Conduct ongoing process and outcome evaluations. In order to ensure the investment in the RWC is well spent, ongoing process and outcome evaluation activities should be conducted to determine

- the penetration of the campaign or the proportion of the intended population the RWC reached and how frequently they were reached
- how the people who were reached compare with the target audiences of the RWC
- how people were exposed to the RWC (e.g., through the website or a brochure, at a conference)
- the impact of the campaign, including what messages and information are salient to users who spend between 13 and 35 seconds on the different sections of the RWC website and what actions people take after being exposed to the RWC materials (e.g., do they access mental health care when it is needed?).

If DCoE is interested in understanding these issues, one option is to embed a small number of questions about the RWC in an existing survey. Questions to assess penetration rate (i.e., the rate at which the RWC is reaching target audiences) should focus on whether individuals have heard of the RWC, whether and how they have accessed and used any of the campaign materials, their perceptions of the quality and believability of the materials, and an assessment of whether the RWC has helped to improve the awareness of mental health issues among servicemembers or helped identify mental health care resources when needed.

There are several ongoing surveys in which DCoE could consider embedding questions about the RWC:

- **Status of Forces Survey.** This survey is conducted annually by the Defense Manpower Data Center. There are separate surveys for active duty, Reserve, and civilian employees. Since 2003, response rates for this survey have been between 28 and 40 percent for active duty (n=~40,000), 25 and 42 percent for Reserve, and 55 and 64 percent for civilian employees. However, it is important to note that in 2010, the U.S. Government Accountability Office raised concerns about this survey because its sponsors do not regularly conduct a nonresponse analysis to determine whether the survey sample is biased.
- **Air Force Community Assessment.** This survey is conducted every 2 to 2.5 years by the Air Force's Community Action Information Board to provide bases' Integrated Service Delivery working groups with information about work and family life and help for community action plans. In 2008, over 75,000 active duty airmen (71 percent), spouses of active duty airmen (15 percent), reserve airmen (11 percent), and civilians (3 percent) working for the Air Force responded. Another survey was fielded in 2011 and results are pending.
- **TRICARE Beneficiary Survey.** This survey is conducted once per calendar quarter (January, April, July, and October) to a sample of all DoD beneficiaries worldwide by the TRICARE Management Authority via contract to a data collection vendor. In 2003, the sample size was approximately 45,000 and was stratified across type of beneficiary and type of coverage. Response rates for the 2003 survey were estimated to be 21 percent for active duty beneficiaries; 32 percent for active duty family members enrolled in TRICARE Prime; 21 percent for active duty family members not enrolled in TRICARE Prime; 57 percent for retirees and their family members younger than 65 enrolled in TRI-

CARE Prime; 48 percent for retirees and family members younger than 65 not enrolled in TRICARE Prime; and 74 percent for retirees and their family members age 65 or older.

A regular evaluation of outcomes will allow the RWC to determine whether the implementation of its activities is of the highest possible quality and whether these activities are generating expected outcomes. This is particularly important given emerging research that suggests the Health Belief Model on which the RWC is based may be limited because it is based on an objective person making planful choices about treatment based on costs and benefits (Corrigan, Rusch, Ben-Zeev, and Sher, under review). In fact, many health decisions are implicit, potentially occurring outside awareness, and are made in reaction to immediate circumstances rather than being planned out or done after careful weighing of costs and benefits (Corrigan, Rusch, Ben-Zeev, and Sher, under review).

Conclusions

The RWC design and dissemination strategies suggest that the RWC shows promise in its ability to reach its intended target audiences and achieve its goals. The expert ratings indicated that the RWC is generally adhering to best practices for health communication campaigns. However, to be responsive to the evolving needs of the military community, media campaigns like the RWC will need to invest in mechanisms that allow them to be nimble. For example, if the long-term goal of the RWC is to ensure that servicemembers in need seek care for mental health problems, then the campaign will need to be aware of and adapt to barriers to mental health care, which will inevitably shift as the system of care evolves. To remain nimble, the RWC should consider clearly communicating the goals of the campaign on its website and in its materials so that these goals are clear and evident to users and partner organizations, particularly if they change over time; more effectively leveraging the existing network of partner organizations; and conducting ongoing research and regular usability testing. To remain relevant to the evolving needs of servicemembers, the RWC should monitor the needs of the target populations and adjust the campaign activities to meet those needs. An annual review of the goals of the RWC, based on objective data such as the MHAT survey findings, would help ensure that the RWC goals are responsive to the changing needs of the military community, including changes to the barriers that servicemembers face when receiving mental health care. Clarifying which materials are tied to which campaign goals and target populations could help the RWC revamp materials quickly as goals are updated.

APPENDIX A

Summary Description of Appendixes B through F

For our assessment, we utilized six complementary methods: (1) a search of the peer-reviewed literature, conducted between January and February 2011; (2) an expert panel that developed a checklist of best practices for health communication campaigns (June 2011) and applied a subset of those checklist items to the RWC (August 2011); (3) telephone discussions with RWC partner organizations conducted between April and June 2011; (4) a content analysis of the RWC website (May 2011); (5) an analysis of communication metrics collected by the RWC (January 2011); and (6) a document review and informal discussions with RWC staff (ongoing between January and August 2011).

In the main body of the report we synthesized the findings from all six of our data sources, since multiple data sources contributed to each aim of the study. These aims are the following:

1. Document the design (goals, target populations, and core messages) and content of the RWC and how the content is disseminated to target populations.
2. Identify the strengths of the content, design, and dissemination strategies used by the RWC and which aspects of the campaign adhere to best practices for health communication campaigns.
3. Identify where DoD should target future investments or quality improvement efforts related to the RWC.

Appendixes B through F summarize the methods and findings for each of the first five data sources. The literature review informed the dialogue and recommendations of the expert panel. The interviews with partner organizations were used to inform our assessment of the breadth of dissemination efforts and elicit the recommendations from partner organizations. The content analysis was used primarily to assess the extent to which the design of the campaign is actually reflected in its content. The communication metrics were primarily used to assess the dissemination of the campaign. Document review and discussions with RWC staff were used to provide the description of the RWC on which this assessment is based.

APPENDIX B

Literature Review Methods and Findings

This appendix describes the methods and findings used in the literature review to identify best practices for health communication campaigns. The appendix concludes with a list of the references reviewed as part of the literature review.

Literature Review Methods

We conducted a search of the peer-reviewed literature to identify best practices and the empirically defined characteristics and qualities of effective behavioral health media campaigns. We reviewed the past 11 years of peer-reviewed research, focusing on citations published in English from January 2000 until February 2011. Multiple databases (PubMed [including MEDLINE], PsycINFO, Web of Science, Defense Technical Information Center, and the ProQuest Military Collection) were used to identify citations using the following key word search strategy:

- Category 1: Keywords specific to barriers or stigma
  - stigma*
  - stigmatize*
  - self-stigma*
  - barrier*
  - access
- Category 2: Keywords specific to media campaigns
  - media
  - messag*
  - communicat*
  - market*
  - campaign*
  - intervention*
  - "social network"
  - "social networks"
  - "social networking"
  - facebook
- Category 3: Keywords specific to mental health or traumatic brain injury
  - mental
  - stress
  - anxiety

  - suicide
  - suicidal depression
  - depressive
  - ptsd
  - mental health services
  - post traumatic stress
  - suicid*
  - combat stress*
- Category 4: Keywords specific to traumatic brain injury
  - TBI
  - traumatic brain injur*
  - brain

  * denotes wildcard search term.

These keywords were identified through a series of test searches to determine which keywords identified the most relevant literature without being overly restrictive. The 256 citations identified by our search strategy underwent a thorough abstract review. Two RAND staff examined titles and abstracts to exclude articles that were not relevant to the task. Articles were included if they described promising, best, or evidence-based practices related to the development or implementation of a media campaign. Articles were excluded if they were published in a language other than English, were focused solely on individuals younger than 18 years old, or were discussion papers, commentaries, letters to the editor, or conference abstracts. We excluded 175 articles during an initial title review using the inclusion/exclusion criteria described above. Next, we reviewed the full abstracts for 81 articles. During the abstract review, an additional 60 articles were excluded. Ultimately, 21 articles met the inclusion criteria and underwent full text review (these citations are listed below). We also examined 14 evaluation reports, working papers, and toolkits identified through feedback from expert panelists and Internet searches published in the gray literature as a way to supplement our examination of the peer-reviewed literature.

We created a data abstraction form (DAF) to facilitate a systematic evaluation of each study reviewed. The DAF captured several items, including source and type of study and media campaign content. We also recorded information from each study that described lessons learned or best practices for designing, formatting, and disseminating a media campaign. RAND staff conducted a pilot test of the DAF to ensure that all researchers were abstracting information in the same way, and the articles were subsequently divided among the team for full review. Counts from the DAFs (source and type of study) are summarized in Table B.1.

Findings from the Literature Review

In this section, we present a summary of the lessons learned and best practices identified in our literature review. The literature review is organized by content area, beginning with practices that should be used during the design of a health communication campaign, followed by practices targeting campaign dissemination. It is important to note that the literature did not

Table B.1
Descriptive Information About Literature Reviewed

	Total Number Reviewed (n=35)
Source	
Peer-reviewed literature	21
Gray literature (e.g., websites, working papers)	14
Content of media campaign	
Mental health	18
Traumatic brain injury	1
Alcohol, tobacco, or other drugs	6
General health	6
Other[a]	4
Type of article	
Evaluation of a media campaign	14
Summary of literature	14
Other[b]	7

[a] Includes campaigns targeted at specific physical health conditions such diabetes or heart disease, as well as campaigns targeting changes in specific business practices.

[b] Includes articles that describe the development of media campaign communication metrics, as well as conceptual and strategic plans.

provide clear guidance about what specific messages are effective in promoting help-seeking behavior, suggesting instead that effective media campaigns tailor messages to specific populations based on age, gender, and other characteristics. This literature and the feedback from the expert panel were utilized to create the final checklist on best practices in health communication campaigns used in the assessment of the RWC, which is shown in Table C.1.

Theoretical Basis

A health communication campaign must have a theory to support its development, and the same theory should serve as a basis for its implementation (e.g., to help define goals and objectives). Before designing campaign materials, developers must conduct thorough research to identify the knowledge, attitudes, and behaviors of target audiences, as well as the behavioral theory that best motivates specific audiences to change (Office on Smoking and Health, 2007; White House Office of National Drug Control Policy, 2011). Theories provide critical information on the determinants of behavior (such as thoughts and feelings) that could potentially lead to the campaign's desired outcomes. Basing a campaign on theory helps developers determine appropriate messages and vehicles on which to place messages (Coffman, 2002; Noar, 2006).

When selecting a theory, the campaign must ensure that it matches the campaign audience (White House Office of National Drug Control Policy, 2011). Research efforts should also identify contextual variables that can affect communications success so that these can be factored into planning (Coffman, 2002; Coffman, 2004). Common research activities during this phase include literature reviews, expert consultation, and review of existing data on the campaign's target population (e.g., demographic and vital statistics).

A theory will also help to guide campaign goals and outcomes. To be effective, the goals and outcomes of campaign communications must be well defined and measurable and must guide a defined plan of action (Coffman, 2004). Given that campaigns are focused, time-bound efforts, campaign activities must closely align with stated goals (Evans-Lacko, London, et al., 2010).

Linkage with Complementary Efforts

To maximize its impact, a health communication campaign must be linked with broader complementary efforts. Research suggests that the campaign's impact is maximized if it is combined with other interventions and strategies, including grassroots promotions, local media advocacy, event sponsorships, and other community tie-ins (Office on Smoking and Health, 2007; Phillipson, Jones, et al., 2009). For example, research has found that pairing media campaigns targeting the stigmatization of homelessness and mental disorders with personal contact from a person who has experienced those issues increased the campaign's effectiveness (Faigin and Stein, 2008; Corrigan, Rafacz, et al., 2010). These linkages help create a network of organizations that both align with and reinforce the campaign messages, creating the supportive environment needed to change a community's prevailing attitudes on the issues the campaign is addressing (Coffman, 2004).

Partner organizations can also add to the credibility and reach of campaign messages (Coffman, 2002). Likewise, negative opinions of these organizations, particularly those who provide services, could hinder mental health care-seeking (McFall, Malte, et al., 2000).

Targeted, Simple, and Clear Messages

Targeting messages to specific homogenous audiences helps focus messages so they are simple and clear. For example, the needs of young people at high risk of mental health problems may be very different from the needs of young people in general, and the preferred style of messages may be very different for young adults and older adults. Evidence suggests that targeting messages to specific audiences can improve their effectiveness (Corrigan and Gelb, 2006). Such targeting will help ensure that messages are framed in ways that are culturally appropriate, reflect audience values, and are relevant and resonate with the target audience (Noar, 2006). Identifying a specific homogenous audience will also help determine the types of messengers that will be seen as credible by the target audiences (Corrigan and Gelb, 2006).

Target Audience Input

The target audiences must have input into the development of campaign messages and strategies for dissemination. A health communication campaign should engage the target audiences early in the campaign development. Input from the target audiences (e.g., through focus groups) should be used to help identify and develop messages that will be relevant to them (Noar, 2006). For example, research has found that messages to encourage help-seeking behavior in men with depression are different from those for women. Although stigma is an important barrier to be addressed for both sexes, self-stigma, or the perception of oneself as inadequate or weak if one were to seek professional help, is particularly salient for men (Hammer and Vogel, 2010). Through this type of formative research, Pietrzak et al. (2009) found that educating servicemembers about the nature and effectiveness of psychological interventions may help decrease stigma and promote help-seeking behaviors.

Health communication campaign developers should also seek input from target audiences about effective dissemination strategies. Various audiences may best be reached through different modes of communication. For example, some researchers suggest that distributing materials through primary care providers is an effective way to reach men with depression (Hammer and Vogel, 2010). Research has also shown that help-seeking messages may be well received by men with depression if those messages are delivered by peers (e.g., those from a similar occupation) or male figures in the public eye (Andreasen, 1994; Rochlen and Hoyer, 2005; Rochlen, McKelley, et al., 2006).

Pilot Test Messages Before Developing or Disseminating

It is critical to rigorously test key messages before investing in the design and development of campaign materials (ads, brochures, public service announcements) and to engage in early pilot tests once materials have been developed. Before developing new campaign materials, developers must identify key messages and then use rigorous qualitative and quantitative testing to ensure that those messages will be effective when they reach their target audiences (White House Office of National Drug Control Policy, 2011).

Research has shown that for messages to be effective they must include a solution or course of action; be simple, clear, and specific to ensure that the audience understands the solution or steps needed to pursue the course of action; and appeal to emotion (Dorfman, Ervice, et al., 2002; Hammer and Vogel, 2010). For example, the Office on Smoking and Health (2007) found that ads with strong negative emotional appeal or that use personal-testimony or graphic-depiction formats can be emotionally engaging and can produce more significant recall among target audiences. The suggested solution or course of action itself must also be well received by the target audience. Some research suggests, for example, that support groups may not be a preferred solution for men with mental health issues (Blazina and Marks, 2001).

Once campaign materials have been developed, they should be pilot tested with the target audiences to assess whether they have the intended impact (Noar, 2006). For example, the National Youth Anti-Drug Media Campaign, *Above the Influence*, shows pilot ads to approximately 300 members of the target audience to assess the ability of the ads to strengthen anti-drug beliefs and attitudes; the ad viewers are compared with a control group whose members do not view the ads. To be selected for use by the National Youth Anti-Drug Media Campaign, each ad must significantly strengthen anti-drug beliefs and attitudes in the test group compared with the matched control group that does not view the ad (White House Office of National Drug Control Policy, 2011). The practice of message testing is based on advertising and market research best practices outlined by leading organizations, such as the American Association for Public Opinion Research, the Advertising Research Foundation, and the Council of American Survey Research Organizations.

Continuous Monitoring and Evaluation

Implementation of a campaign should be accompanied by continuous monitoring and evaluation. Assessing whether the campaign is having its intended impact can help inform mid-course corrections if a campaign is not achieving its goals and objectives, as well as modifications needed for a campaign to stay current (Noar, 2006). Additionally, campaigns must be evaluated to investigate whether they have been successful in changing behaviors and attitudes or in meeting other goals. For example, the National Youth Anti-Drug Media Campaign surveys 100 teens every week to assess how their ads are performing, measuring teen awareness and memory of ads as well as teen attitudes about drugs and intentions regarding drug use. Additionally, the National Youth Anti-Drug Media Campaign surveys 100 parents of teens each week to assess the parent-focused ads (White House Office of National Drug Control Policy, 2011). Building evaluation activities into any campaign, at any level, ensures that resources are not wasted (Noar, 2006).

Regular and Consistent Message Exposure

A campaign must maintain a strong and consistent presence in media accessed by the target audiences. A typical pattern of audience reaction to health communication campaigns is to first notice, then internalize, and then react to messages (e.g., change of attitudes or behaviors) (Pinfold, Thornicroft, et al., 2005). Health communication campaigns should feature multiple message strategies and media channels to consistently attract, engage, and influence their target populations. To effectively reach target audiences, campaign developers should rely on media outlets utilized by their target audiences. For example, the Internet may be an important outlet for younger cohorts who are spending more time on the Internet and playing video games (Television Bureau of Advertising, 2008). It is also important to note that the optimal mix of media outlets depends on the size of the available budget. A 2003 study of advertising found that print, radio, or television advertising was the preferred medium at low, medium, and high budget levels, respectively (Dertouzos, Polich, et al., 1989; Dertouzos and Garber, 2003).

Outreach and dissemination to audiences through multiple outlets should be regular and sustained to ensure adequate exposure to and retention of campaign messages (Phillipson, Jones, et al., 2009). Research suggests that, before it is launched, a health communication campaign should strategically plan to reach 75 percent to 85 percent of the target audience every three months during the life of the campaign, with a more concentrated effort during the first three to six months (Office on Smoking and Health, 2007).

Advertising industry standards use a targeted rating point as an indicator of whether a campaign has had the reach and frequency required to have an impact (Evans-Lacko, London, et al., 2010). Targeted rating points are calculated by multiplying the reach of a campaign (i.e., the unduplicated percentage of the target population who saw the campaign) by the frequency (how many times the campaign was viewed by the target population). During the initial three to six months of a campaign, industry standards suggest that the campaign should maintain an average of 1,200 targeted rating points per quarter and 800 targeted rating points per quarter thereafter (Office on Smoking and Health, 2007). It is critical for health communication campaigns to include a strategic plan for reaching the necessary targeted rating points. Exposure to a health communication campaign does not automatically equal success (Rochlen, Whilde, et al., 2005). The target audience must pay attention to the health communication campaign with enough frequency to be able to recognize and recall campaign messages. A campaign should be expected to run at least six months to affect awareness of the issue, 12 to 18 months to have an impact on attitudes, and 18 to 24 months to influence behavior (Office on Smoking and Health, 2007).

Mental Health Communication Campaigns Targeting Male Audiences

Health communication campaigns targeting mental health issues among men have unique considerations. Hammer and Vogel (2010) found that tailoring materials to men by using language more compatible with traditional gender roles (e.g., "team up," "tackle the problem," "defeat depression") improved their effectiveness in reducing the self-stigma associated with seeking mental health counseling. Likewise, other research has shown that messages targeting mental health issues among men, particularly depression, should emphasize that professional help will support strong, healthy, autonomous decisionmaking (Andreasen, 1994; Rochlen and Hoyer, 2005); discuss the symptoms most associated with depression in men such as substance use, aggression, and withdrawal (Rochlen, McKelley, et al., 2006; Hammer and Vogel, 2010); provide evidence for treatment as a cost-effective endeavor (Rochlen, McKelley, et al., 2006; Hammer and Vogel, 2010); and highlight the biological underpinnings of depression to counter the misperception that mental illnesses such as depression stem from lack of willpower (Hammer and Vogel, 2010).

References Cited in the Literature Review

Andreasen, A. R. (1994). "Social marketing: Definition and domain." *Journal of Marketing and Public Policy* **13**: 108–114.

Blazina, C., and L. I. Marks (2001). "College men's affective reactions to individual therapy, psychoeducational workshops, and men's support group brochures: The influence of gender-role conflict and power dynamics upon help-seeking attitudes." *Psychotherapy* **38**(3): 297–305.

Coffman, J. (2002). *Public Communication Campaign Evaluation: An Environmental Scan of Challenges, Criticisms, Practice, and Opportunities.* Cambridge, MA: Harvard Family Research Project.

Coffman, J. (2004). *Strategic Communications Audits.* Washington, DC: Communications Consortium Media Center.

Corrigan, P., and B. Gelb (2006). "Three programs that use mass approaches to challenge the stigma of mental illness." *Psychiatric Services* **57**(3): 393–398.

Corrigan, P. W., J. D. Rafacz, et al. (2010). "Changing stigmatizing perceptions and recollections about mental illness: the effects of NAMI's In Our Own Voice." *Community Mental Health Journal* **46**(5): 517–522.

Dertouzos, J., and S. Garber (2003). *Is Military Advertising Effective? An Estimation of Methodology and Applications to Recruiting in the 1980s and 90s.* Santa Monica, CA: RAND Corporation.

Dertouzos, J., J. M. Polich, A. Bamezai, and T. W. Chesnutt (1989). *Recruiting Effects of Army Advertising.* Santa Monica, CA: RAND Corporation.

Dorfman, L., J. Ervice, et al. (2002). *Voices for Change: A Taxonomy of Public Communications Campaigns and Their Evaluation Challenges.* Berkeley, CA: Berkeley Media Studies Group.

Evans-Lacko, S., J. London, et al. (2010). "Evaluation of a brief anti-stigma campaign in Cambridge: Do short-term campaigns work?" *BMC Public Health* **10**: 339.

Faigin, D. A., and C. H. Stein (2008). "Comparing the effects of live and video-taped theatrical performance in decreasing stigmatization of people with serious mental illness." *Journal of Mental Health* **17**(6): 594–606.

Hammer, J. H., and D. L. Vogel (2010). "Men's help seeking for depression: The efficacy of a male-sensitive brochure about counseling." *The Counseling Psychologist* **38**(2): 296–313.

McFall, M., C. Malte, et al. (2000). "Effects of an outreach intervention on use of mental health services by veterans with posttraumatic stress disorder." *Psychiatric Services* **51**(3): 369–374.

Noar, S. M. (2006). "A 10-year retrospective of research in health mass media campaigns: Where do we go from here?" *Journal of Health Communication* **11**(1): 21–42.

Office on Smoking and Health (2007). *Best Practices for Comprehensive Tobacco Control Programs—2007: Section A: Health Communications Interventions.* Atlanta, GA: U.S. Department of Health and Human Services, Centers for Disease Control and Prevention, National Center for Chronic Disease Prevention and Health Promotion.

Phillipson, L., S. Jones, et al. (2009). "Effective communication only part of the strategy needed to promote help-seeking of young people with mental health problems." *Social Marketing Quarterly* **15**(2): 50–62.

Pietrzak, R. H., D. C. Johnson, M. B. Goldstein, J. C. Malley, and S. M. Southwick (2009). "Perceived stigma and barriers to mental health care utilization among OEF-OIF veterans." *Psychiatric Services* **60**(8): 1118–1122.

Pinfold, V. G., G. Thornicroft, et al. (2005). "Active ingredients in anti-stigma programmes in mental health." *International Review of Psychiatry* **17**(2): 123–131.

Rochlen, A. B., and W. D. Hoyer (2005). "Marketing mental health to men: Theoretical and practical considerations." *Journal of Clinical Psychology* **61**(6): 675–684.

Rochlen, A. B., R. A. McKelley, et al. (2006). "A preliminary examination of the 'Real Men. Real Depression' campaign." *Psychology of Men and Masculinity* 7(1): 1–13.

Rochlen, A., M. Whilde, et al. (2005). "The Real Men. Real Depression campaign: Overview, theoretical implications, and research considerations." *Psychology of Men and Masculinity* **63**(3): 186–194.

Television Bureau of Advertising (2008). *2008 Media Comparisons Study.* New York, NY: Nielsen Media Research.

White House Office of National Drug Control Policy (2011). National Youth Anti-Drug Media Campaign.

APPENDIX C

Expert Panel Methods and Findings

This appendix describes how we convened the expert panel and who the expert panelists were, as well as the process used by the expert panelists to develop the final checklist of best practices for health communication campaigns based on the literature review described in Appendix B. The final checklist of best practices for health communication campaigns is shown in Table C.1.

Expert Panel Methods

Experts participated in a two-phase process to develop a checklist of best practices in health communication campaigns and then to apply a subset of items from the checklist to the RWC.

Convening the Expert Panel

We convened a panel consisting of ten experts in five key areas:

- barriers to mental health care, including stigma
- mental health in the military (PTSD, deployment psychology)
- effective media campaigns
- media campaigns for servicemembers
- psychological resilience.

The experts that served on the panel in each of these five areas were the following:

Area 1: Experts on Barriers to Mental Health Care, Including Stigma

Howard Goldman, M.D., Ph.D., is Professor of Psychiatry at the University of Maryland School of Medicine and is currently the director of the Network on Mental Health Policy Research. Dr. Goldman also acted as Senior Scientific Editor of the Surgeon General's Report on Mental Health (1997–1999) and consultant to the President's New Freedom Commission on Mental Health (2002–2003).

Aaron Rochlen, Ph.D., is an Associate Professor of Counseling and Educational Psychology at the University of Texas in Austin. Dr. Rochlen specializes in the study of men's gender role socialization and help-seeking behaviors and the potential of alternative marketing approaches and counseling techniques for men. He also served as lead evaluator of the "Real Men. Real Depression" media campaign.

Area 2: Expert on Mental Health in the Military (PTSD, deployment psychology)

Harold Kudler, Ph.D., is Associate Clinical Professor at Duke University and coordinates mental health services for a three-state region of the VA. Dr. Kudler has also served as co-chair of the VA's Special Committee on PTSD.

Area 3: Experts on Effective Media Campaigns

Rebecca Collins, Ph.D., heads the Program on Health Promotion and Disease Prevention within RAND Health. Dr. Collins' research focuses on the effects of media on adolescent development. She currently leads an ongoing national longitudinal study testing associations between television viewing and adolescent sexual attitudes and behavior.

Cynthia Bauer, Ph.D., is the Director of Health Communication and Marketing for the National Center for Health Marketing, operated by the Centers for Disease Control and Prevention.

Area 4: Experts on Media Campaigns for Servicemembers

Deborah Leiter is a campaign manager at the Ad Council, the leading producer of public service announcements.

Nancy Vineburgh, M.A., is an Assistant Professor in the Department of Psychiatry at the Uniformed Services University of the Health Sciences in Bethesda, Maryland, and serves as the Director of the Office of Public Education and Preparedness at the Center for the Study of Traumatic Stress. Ms. Vineburgh is an expert in health communication, health marketing, and public education and has created numerous, high-profile public education campaigns (e.g., Courage to Care, an electronic campaign addressing the well-being of deployed servicemembers and their families).

John Parrish, M.D., is the Founder and Executive Director of the Center for Integration of Medicine and Innovative Technology and Director of the Massachusetts General Hospital Home Base Program, a program aimed at helping military veterans affected by PTSD and TBI through outreach and support services.

Area 5: Experts on Psychological Resilience

Brett Litz, Ph.D., is a Professor in the Department of Psychiatry at Boston University School of Medicine and the Psychology Department at Boston University as well as the Associate Director of the Behavioral Sciences Division of the National Center for PTSD at the VA Boston Health Care System. Dr. Litz's research focuses on early intervention strategies for survivors of trauma, including an Internet-based self-management approach to the treatment of PTSD.

Shelley MacDermid, Ph.D., is a Professor in the Department of Child Development and Family Studies at Purdue University, where she also directs the Military Family Research Institute and the Center for Families and serves as Associate Dean of the College of Consumer and Family Sciences.

- the "Partners" link, which provides information on the types of organizations with which the RWC has developed relationships
- the "Resources" link, which lists links to specific resources for specific target populations
- the "Videos" link, which provides public service announcements, video profiles containing servicemember stories, and e-cards developed by the RWC
- the "Campaign Materials" link, which includes the brochures, posters, and web banners developed by the RWC. A web banner is a form of online advertising embedded in a web page (e.g., a partner web page). It is intended to attract traffic to the RWC website.

Panelists were asked to track which material they reviewed (see Tables C.3–C.10).

After the panelists reviewed the RWC website, they were asked to use their best judgment to rate the campaign using the seven checklist items that pertained to the campaign website (Items 1–7). For each checklist item, panel members were asked to provide (1) an overall rating based on their review of the entire website; (2) a rating for each target population based on their review of the materials for that specific target population; and (3) a brief rationale for their rating.

Overall ratings reflected an aggregate impression of the extent to which the RWC adheres to the checklist item based on their review of all the website content, including the sections highlighted above. Experts were able to review the website during the rating process. The rating scale for overall rating ranged from strongly agree (7 = most or all of the website materials you reviewed adhered to the checklist item) to strongly disagree (1 = most or all of the website materials you reviewed did not adhere to the checklist item).

Ratings for each target population were based on a more specific subset of website content tailored for one of the five main target populations: active duty, National Guard and Reserve, veterans, families, and health professionals. Ratings for each target population reflected an aggregate impression of the extent to which the RWC adheres to the checklist item, relying on website sections tailored specifically to that target population. Similar to the overall ratings, the rating scale ranged from strongly agree (7 = most or all of the website materials for that target population adhered to the checklist item) to strongly disagree (1 = most or all of the website materials for that target population did not adhere to the checklist item).

For each rating, panel members were also asked to identify the specific sections of the website or specific campaign resources, partners, videos, and materials that contributed to their decision, and to provide comments on how the RWC can modify and improve its website and materials.

Findings from the Expert Panel Ratings of the Real Warriors Campaign

We found that the expert ratings of the RWC materials varied widely, as evidenced by the ranges in the tables below. In particular, we observed significant disagreement between experts for Items 1 to 5. *Significant disagreement* was defined as ratings from two or more panelists being more than three points away from the other panelists' ratings. To better understand the variation, we convened a panel meeting to discuss the rationale behind the overall website ratings for Items 1 to 5. After the discussion of each item, experts were asked to re-rate the overall website for Items 1 to 5. We display both the initial ratings provided by experts before the meeting and the ratings provided by experts after further discussion of each item during the meeting (the revised ratings). After discussion of each item, ratings tended to decrease.

The overall mean ratings (Table C.2) suggest that the RWC materials generally adhere to the best practices for health communication campaigns that are included in the checklist. However, even after re-rating, experts significantly disagreed on whether the RWC materials clearly communicate the messages of the campaign and are simple enough to be easily understood, and whether the messages convey a solution or clear course of action. Expert ratings most strongly converged on ratings regarding the RWC messengers being seen as credible to the active duty target audience, but did not agree as to whether the RWC messengers would be seen as credible among other target audiences, including National Guard and Reserve servicemembers, veterans, families, and health professionals. Experts also strongly agreed that RWC avoids reinforcing negative stereotypes.

Tables C.3–C.10 display a summary of the website content that each expert panel member reviewed to rate the RWC materials. Each table represents a separate section of the website. One expert was not able to complete a review of the website during the specified timeframe for reasons unrelated to this evaluation. As a result, the ratings in these tables are listed for only nine of the ten panelists.

Table C.2
Expert Panel Ratings of the Real Warriors Campaign (Mean, Range)

	Items from the Checklist of Best Practices for Health Communication Campaigns						
	RWC materials . . .		RWC messages . . .			RWC . . .	
Website section	Clearly communicate the messages of the campaign	Are simple enough to be easily understood	Are simple and clear	Convey a solution or clear course of action	Are compelling	Messengers will be seen as credible to the target audience of the RWC	Avoids reinforcing negative stereotypes
Overall website (initial rating)	4.7, 3–6	4.8, 3–7	5.6, 3–7	4.6, 3–6	4.4, 2–6	6.5, 5–7	6.1, 5–7
Overall website (revised rating)	3.8, 2–6	3.8, 2–6	5.2, 3–7	3.9, 2–6	4.1, 2–5	—[a]	—[a]
Active duty	4.8, 3–7	5.4, 3–7	5.0, 3–7	4.6, 3–6	4.6, 2–6	6.4, 5–7	6.3, 6–7
National Guard and Reserve	4.3, 1–7	4.9, 2–7	4.8, 3–7	4.2, 1–6	4.2, 1–6	5.9, 1–7	5.9, 3–7
Veterans	4.8, 3–7	5.3, 3–7	4.9, 3–7	4.3, 2–6	4.7, 2–7	6.0, 1–7	6.1, 4–7
Families[b]	4.8, 3–7	5.6, 3–7	5.1, 3–7	4.4, 2–7	4.3, 2–6	5.8, 1–7	5.9, 2–7
Health professionals	4.3, 2–6	5.6, 2–7	4.6, 1–7	4.6, 2–7	4.4, 2–6	5.3, 1–7	6.3, 4–7

[a] These items were not re-rated because there was no significant disagreement on their initial rating.

[b] Families include caregivers, adolescents, and children.

Table C.3
Summary of the Active Duty Section of the Website Reviewed by Expert Panelists to Inform Their Ratings of the Real Warriors Campaign

	Panelist								
Active Duty Section of the Website	**1**	**2**	**3**	**4**	**5**	**6**	**7**	**8**	**9**
Building Resilience as an Individual Augmentee	x	x	x		x	x		x	
Developing Healthy Sleeping Habits While Deployed	x		x			x	x		
Prepare for the Challenges of Multiple Deployments			x				x		
Preparing for Deployment		x	x	x	x	x		x	x
Combat Stress: A Natural Result of Heavy Mental and Emotional Work		x	x				x		x
Nutrition's Role in Building Resilience			x			x	x	x	x
Physical Fitness Training Year-Round Boost Resilience			x		x	x		x	
Behavioral Fitness: Coping Skills Build Resilience			x					x	
Boosting Resilience Through Spirituality			x		x		x		
Dispelling Myths About Post-Traumatic Stress Disorder			x	x	x	x	x	x	x
Social Fitness: Building Health Social Ties			x						
Psychological Fitness–Keeping Your Mind Fit			x		x				
Dealing with Depression: Symptoms and Treatment			x		x	x	x	x	x
Monitor Psychological Health with the T2 Mood Tracker App			x						
Free Support Program for Warriors in Transition									
Strategies for Managing Stress at Events			x		x				x
You Are Not Alone: Suicide Prevention Tools for Warriors	x		x	x	x				x
Cognitive Rehabilitation Helps Warriors with Mild TBI					x		x		
Maintain Family Strength When Both Parents Deploy					x				
Get Help Online with TRICARE's New Assistance Program					x				x
No Ordinary Warrior: Your Chaplain Is a Frontline Resource					x	x	x		
Maintaining Psychological Strength While Deployed			x					x	
Build Resilience to Maximize Readiness		x	x	x				x	
Traumatic Brain Injury: Signs and Symptoms					x			x	x
Traumatic Brain Injury: Treatment and Recovery							x	x	x
You Are a Friend's Biggest Support				x	x				x
Disability Evaluation System									
How to Reconnect with Your Teen After Deployment					x	x	x		
8 Battlefield Skills that Make Reintegration Challenging						x		x	
Reintegrating Info Family Life After Deployment					x				
Five Tips to Reinforce Unit Cohesion			x		x				
Strong Leadership Aids Warrior Resilience			x				x		
Line Leaders Managing Personnel in Distress			x			x			x
Army Resources					x		x		
Navy Resources		x			x		x		
Marine Corps Resources		x	x		x		x		
Air Force Resources		x			x		x		

Table C.4
Summary of the National Guard and Reserve Section of the Website Reviewed by Expert Panelists to Inform Their Ratings of the Real Warriors Campaign

	Panelist								
National Guard and Reserve Section of the Website	**1**	**2**	**3**	**4**	**5**	**6**	**7**	**8**	**9**
Developing Healthy Sleep Patterns While Deployed			x	x	x				
Prepare for the Challenges of Multiple Deployments			x				x		
Preparing for Deployment			x		x				x
Plan for Financial Readiness Before Deployment			x				x		
Reintegrating into Family Life After Deployment			x		x		x		x
8 Battlefield Skills that Make Reintegration Challenging	x		x						
Easing Holiday and Reintegration Stress for Service Members			x						
How to Reconnect with Your Teen After Deployment	x		x				x		x
7 Ways to Thank National Guardsmen and Reservists			x	x	x				
What the Post–9/11 GI Bill Means to You			x		x				
How Guard and Reserve Veterans Get Support From VA			x						
Yellow Ribbon Program: Support for Guard and Reserve			x		x		x		
For Employers: Helping Employees Reintegrate into Civilian Employment			x	x					
For Employees: Reintegrating into Civilian Employment			x						
Reintegrating into Civilian Life		x	x		x		x		
What Line of Duty Determinations Mean to Guard and Reserve Members			x						
You Are Not Alone: Suicide Prevention Tools for Warriors			x						x
Combat Stress: A Natural Result of Heavy Mental Work			x		x				x
Dealing with Depression: Symptoms and Treatment			x				x		x
Build Resilience to Maximize Mission Readiness			x		x				
Maintaining Psychological Strength While Deployed		x	x						
Dispelling Myths About PTSD			x		x		x		x
National Guard Psychological Health Program			x	x					
Outreach Center for Psychological Health and Traumatic Brain Injury Support			x		x		x		
Knowing What the Red Cross Can Do for You			x						
Resources			x	x					

Table C.5
Summary of the Veterans Section of the Website Reviewed by Expert Panelists to Inform Their Ratings of the Real Warriors Campaign

	Panelist								
Veterans Section of the Website	**1**	**2**	**3**	**4**	**5**	**6**	**7**	**8**	**9**
Veterans Affairs in the Digital Age	x				x		x	x	x
Compensation, Pension, and Other VA Benefits							x	x	
Veterans Affairs Health Benefits Overview	x						x		
Applying for Discharge Upgrade					x				
Four Tips to Successfully Manage Chronic Pain					x		x		x
Building Resilience to Cope with Difficult Situations								x	
Translating Military Experience to Civilian Employment				x			x		
Do Something Meaningful for Veterans Day					x				
Managing Stress in the Workplace					x		x	x	x
Vet Centers Provide Reintegration Support for Warriors									
Accessing Benefits for PTSD Is Easier than Ever					x		x		x
Five Resources for Returning to School					x				
How Veterans Can Aid Resilience by Writing							x		
How Veterans Can Address Substance Misuse					x				
Your Post-Military Career: Tips for Finding a Job and Achieving Success in the Civilian Workplace				x					
Five Steps Veterans Can Take to Support PTSD Treatment					x		x	x	x
Resources		x					x	x	

Table C.6
Summary of the Families[a] Section of the Website Reviewed by Expert Panelists to Inform Their Ratings of the Real Warriors Campaign

	Panelist								
Families Section of the Website	**1**	**2**	**3**	**4**	**5**	**6**	**7**	**8**	**9**
Maintaining Relationships with Loved Ones During Deployment		x			x	X	x	x	
Boosting Family Resilience		x		x	x			x	x
Military Family Life Consultants Ease Warrior Transitions							x		
New Parents Can Stay Connected During Deployment				x	x		x	x	
Tips for Spouses of Returning Service Members					x		x	x	x
Domestic Violence Resources for Military Families	x				x				x
Suicide Prevention Resources for Military Families					x		x		x
How Parents of Warriors Can Support Reintegration	x				x			x	
Supporting Your Service Member with Psychological Health Concerns				x			x		
Role of Family and Loved Ones in Substance Misuse					x				
Strengthen Your Family with Marital Counseling		x							
Caring for Yourself While Helping Support Your Service Member					x		x	x	x
Helping Children Through the Grieving Process		x			x	x			
Teens & Deployment: What to Expect and How to Help					x	x			x
Sesame Workshop Helps Children Cope with Grief		x				x	x	x	x
April Is the Month of the Military Child						x		x	
Preparing Children For Deployment		x						x	x
Taking Care of You—Taking Care of Your Children						x	x		x
Transitioning Through a Reunion						x			x
Talk, Listen, Connect—A Family Focused Initiative for the Military Community					x	x	x		x
Resources		x			x		x	x	

[a] Families include caregivers, adolescents, and children.

Table C.7
Summary of the Health Professionals Section of the Website Reviewed by Expert Panelists to Inform Their Ratings of the Real Warriors Campaign

	Panelist								
Health Professionals Section of the Website	**1**	**2**	**3**	**4**	**5**	**6**	**7**	**8**	**9**
How to Become a TRICARE Accepting Provider	x	x			x	x	x		x
Post-Deployment CPG Desk Reference Toolbox		x				x	x		x
Understanding and Using Evidence-Based Clinical Practice Guidelines		x	x	x	x	x	x		x
Building Resilience for Military Health Professionals			x		x			x	
Tools to Use when Counseling Service Members	x			x			x	x	
Online Learning for Health Professionals				x	x	x	x	x	
National Resource Directory: 10,000 Services and Resources							x		
Resources		x			x		x	x	

Table C.8
Summary of the Partners Section of the Website by Expert Panelists to Inform Their Ratings of the Real Warriors Campaign

	Panelist								
Partners Section of the Website	**1**	**2**	**3**	**4**	**5**	**6**	**7**	**8**	**9**
DCoE Component Centers	x				x	x	x		x
Federal and Military Organizations					x		x		
National Organizations				x			x		
Local Organizations	x								x

Table C.9
Summary of the Campaign Materials Section of the Website Reviewed by Expert Panelists to Inform Their Ratings of the Real Warriors Campaign

	Panelist								
Campaign Materials Section of the Website	**1**	**2**	**3**	**4**	**5**	**6**	**7**	**8**	**9**
Real Warriors Brochure		x		x	x	x	x	x	x
Real Warriors Campaign Brochure for National Guard and Reserve		x		x	x				
Real Warriors Campaign Brochure for Military Families		x		x	x		x	x	
Real Warriors Overview		x		x	x			x	x
Real Warriors Backgrounder		x		x	x		x		
Campaign Ads and Posters: Marine Corps 1	x	x		x	x			x	x
Campaign Ads and Posters: Marine Corps 2					x				
Campaign Ads and Posters: Army 1		x		x	x		x		x
Campaign Ads and Posters: Army 2					x				
Campaign Ads and Posters: Navy 1	x	x		x	x		x		
Campaign Ads and Posters: Navy 2					x				
Campaign Ads and Posters: Air Force 1				x	x				
Campaign Ads and Posters: Air Force 2				x	x		x		
Real Warriors Campaign Web Banners					x				

Table C.10
Summary of the Videos Section of the Website Reviewed by Expert Panelists to Inform Their Ratings of the Real Warriors Campaign

	Panelist								
Videos Section of the Website	**1**	**2**	**3**	**4**	**5**	**6**	**7**	**8**	**9**
Video Profiles									
Real Warriors and Psychological Health		x		x	x		x	x	x
SSgt Stacy Pearsall	x	x			x			x	x
Real Warriors and Resilience					x			x	
Real Warriors					x				
Capt Joshua Mantz					x			x	x
Maj Ed Pulido					x		x		
Real Warriors and Families					x			x	
Lt Col Mary Carlise		x			x				
Maj Jeff Hall	x				x			x	
SSgt Megan Krause					x		x		
Capt Emily Stehr					x				
From the Hearts of Heroes: Thoughts About Combat Stress					x			x	
Maj Gen David Blackledge				x	x				
Maj Iwona Blackledge					x				
SSgt Josh Hopper					x		x	x	
Video PSAs									
Maj Ed Pulido		x	x		x			x	x
Emmitt Smith and Jerome Bettis	x	x		x	x				
Hearts of Heroes (29 seconds)		x		x	x			x	
Hearts of Heroes (59 seconds)				x	x			x	
Capt Josh Mantz		x		x			x		x
Capt Josh Mantz and Maj Ed Pulido					x		x	x	x
Vet Centers		x			x				
Richard "Mack" Manchowicz			x						
Eric Hipple and Capt Mark McNeill					x				
SSgt Megan Krause (29 seconds)					x	x	x		
SSgt Megan Krause (59 seconds)					x				
Maj Jeff Hall (29 seconds)					x			x	
Maj Jeff Hall (59 seconds)					x			x	
Sgt Josh Hopper (29 seconds)					x		x	x	
Sgt Josh Hopper (59 seconds)					x			x	
Voices (29 seconds)									
Voices (59 seconds)									
Radio PSAs									
Real Warriors Reaching Out									x
Real Warriors and Families							x		
Capt Mark McNeill and Eric Hipple	x				x				

Table C.10—Continued

	Panelist								
Videos Section of the Website	**1**	**2**	**3**	**4**	**5**	**6**	**7**	**8**	**9**
E-cards									
Air Force				x		x	x		x
Army									x
Marines							x		
Navy				x					
Coast Guard									
Families	x						x		x

APPENDIX D

Discussions with Real Warriors Campaign Partner Organizations

This appendix describes how we identified and recruited partner organizations for telephone discussions, how we conducted the partner discussions, and the key themes we identified from a qualitative analysis of the discussions. It concludes with a full list of all RWC partner organizations.

Methods Used for Partner Discussions

Our telephone discussions with partner organizations assessed how the campaign has been disseminated and determined partner organizations' perceptions of the campaign and its materials. Local, national, and military organizations and DCoE component centers all partner with the campaign to disseminate materials through announcements, articles, blogs, and other links to their websites. RAND researchers talked with a sample of these partner organizations to determine how they are partnering with the campaign and using campaign materials and to assess their perceptions of the utility and effectiveness of those materials.

Identifying and Recruiting Partner Organizations

RWC staff provided us with an initial list of their partner organizations as of December 2010 and an updated list as of July 2011. A list of the RWC's 153 partners is included at the end of this appendix. The list included information about the partner organizations' roles in relation to the campaign, the primary strategic purpose guiding each organization's partnership with the RWC, and which entity initiated the partner relationship (i.e., RWC or the partner organization). To learn more about the partner organizations, we searched their websites for information concerning their target populations, primary mission and activities, and type of organization (e.g., educational institution, government organization), and noted the location of the RWC web link and/or logo on each partnering organization's website. Using the most up-to-date information available at the time of recruitment, we selected a sample of 35 of the RWC's partner organizations, with an expectation that at least 70 percent (n = 25) would participate in discussions. We purposively selected the sample to include a diverse cross-section of organizations based on both the information provided by the RWC and the information gathered by RAND staff while searching partner organizations' websites.

RWC staff informed key leaders (e.g., program managers and directors) at these 35 partner organizations about the study via email prior to recruitment. RAND staff then emailed and/or telephoned these key leaders to schedule telephone discussions with them or their designated staff members. Twenty-six individuals, each representing a different organization, chose to participate. We reviewed the final sample to confirm that it included a diverse cross-section of organizations, based on both the information provided by the RWC and the information gathered by RAND staff while searching partner organizations' websites (Table D.1). For example, we purposely included a variety of types of partners so that we had at least one

Table D.1
Characteristics of Partner Organizations (n = 26)

	No.
Initiation	
Campaign initiated contact with partner	20
Partner initiated contact with campaign	6
Strategic Purpose(s) of Partnership with the RWC[a]	
Create awareness about mental health concerns	23
Increase stakeholder knowledge of resources available	26
Facilitate access to care or remove barriers to care	23
Other, including involvement in campaign launch or serving as a local resource	9
Role(s) as Partner[a]	
Lists the campaign logo and/or web link on partner's website	21
Publishes articles or news briefs about the campaign	12
Includes campaign updates in e-blasts, e-newsletters, social media and/or blogs	14
Disseminates or displays campaign materials (e.g., at events or in offices or clinics)	15
Is listed as a resource in the partner section of RWC website	26
Is listed as a resource in articles on the RWC website	13
Other, including conferences, roundtables, and briefings	5
Target Population(s)[a]	
Active duty servicemembers	15
National Guard or Reserve	15
Veterans	14
Family members	18
Health professionals	9
Primary Mission and Activities[a]	
Advocacy	6
Communication or media campaign	3
Education and training	2
Readiness and resilience	2
Readjustment and reintegration	6
Recreation	2
Research	3
Resources and information	9
Social support	7
Treatment, care, or care coordination	3
Other, including outreach, employment services, and homeless resources	3

Table D.1—Continued

Organization Type	
Educational or research institution	3
Government agency program: VA	1
Government agency program: DoD	4
Government agency program: other	1
Professional association	1
Veterans Service Organization (VSO)	4
Other not-for-profit organization	12

[a] Categories are not mutually exclusive.

research institution, one government agency program, one professional association, one veterans' service organization, and one nonprofit organization. Similarly we purposely selected partners that served a variety of target populations (e.g., veterans, family members, servicemembers) and represented a range of missions or primary activities (e.g., advocacy, care, education).

Collecting and Analyzing Partner Discussions

Between April and June 2011, we conducted 30-minute individual telephone discussions with key staff at the 26 partner organizations that responded to our recruiting efforts. Discussions covered partner organizations' goals and activities; constituents served; modes of communication with constituents; modes of engagement with the RWC; utilization of RWC materials; perceptions of the utility and effectiveness of these materials; and recommendations for improving the RWC. Notes were taken during each discussion and used for analysis.

We conducted a qualitative analysis in accordance with grounded theory (Glaser and Strauss, 1967; Strauss and Corbin, 1998), an established methodology for systematically analyzing qualitative data. To do so, we followed four key steps:

1. **Identifying codes.** We read through the discussion notes to examine phrases and sentences and generate codes that described them.
2. **Identifying themes.** After categorizing and sorting the data using codes, we clustered related codes together into nine thematic categories identified by project staff as appropriate descriptors of the underlying data.
3. **Checking for accuracy and consistency.** Multiple team members reviewed the codes, themes, and discussion notes to ensure the accuracy and consistency of the codes and themes. Any discrepencies were resolved by consensus.
4. **Checking for saturation.** As the discussions neared completion, we reviewed discussion notes to ensure saturation (defined as the point at which holding discussions with additional partners would no longer provide new input about the topics being investigated).

Findings from Partner Discussions

Table D.2 displays a summary of the key themes identified from discussions with partner organizations and the frequency with which they occurred across the 26 discussions.

Table D.2
Frequency of Themes Abstracted from Partner Organization Discussions

Theme	Number of Discussions in Which Theme Was Raised
Need to broaden and deepen partnerships	
Partner organizations would like more interaction with the RWC	14
Partner organizations would like more interaction with other partners	7
Partner organizations would like to be better educated and informed about the RWC	3
Partner organizations would like to be segmented, or clustered by geographic region, target population, or type of services offered	3
Web link traffic from the RWC to its partner organization websites is minimal	2
Partner organizations would like the RWC to deepen its relationships with government agencies	2
Need to clarify and maintain the mission/goals of campaign	
Partner organizations perceive the RWC to be a means for educating and informing their target populations	12
Partner organizations perceive the RWC to be a source for resources and referrals to their services	9
Partner organizations perceive the RWC to be an anti-stigma campaign	7
Partner organizations would like the RWC to add a focus on audiences outside the military	4
Partner organizations would like the RWC to reach out more to military families	3
Partner organizations are conflating the RWC with DCoE	3
Partner organizations have positive feelings about a publication that DCoE released	2
Need to expand the modes of dissemination	
Partner organizations and/or their constituents are utilizing social media	6
Partner organizations would like the RWC to conduct more face-to-face outreach	4
Partner organizations would like the RWC to have more presence at events and conferences	4
Partner organizations view mobile technologies as an area that the RWC should further explore	3
Partner organizations are featuring the RWC in their newsletter	2
Lack feedback mechanisms	
Partner organizations feel that the RWC is disseminating materials without gathering feedback	10
Mixed feedback about materials	
Partner organizations have positive feelings about the RWC materials	7
Partner organizations report not using the RWC materials	3
Partner organizations report that their constituents are "pamphleted to death," or provided with too many print materials	2
Partner organizations report that the RWC materials need improving	2
Partner organizations report wanting more RWC materials	2
Need more than a campaign	
Partner organizations feel that the RWC could do more to provide "warm handoffs" or connect its target populations to local resources	2
Partner organizations are questioning the overall usefulness of the RWC	2
Partner organizations perceive that concerns about the health care system, rather than stigma, are the primary barriers to care	2

Table D.2—Continued

Theme	Number of Discussions in Which Theme Was Raised
Need targeted, streamlined messaging	
Partner organizations would like the RWC messaging to be more relevant to the RWC target populations	6
Partner organizations would like the RWC to simplify its messaging	4
Partner organizations would like the RWC to avoid mention of mental illness in its messaging	2
Positive feedback about videos, with improvement suggestions	
Partner organizations have positive feelings about the video PSAs	10
Partner organizations would like more older-generation veterans to be portrayed in video PSAs	3
Partner organizations would like others such as caregivers, the homeless, and junior enlisted personnel to be portrayed in video PSAs	3
Partner organizations would like more women to be portrayed in video PSAs	2
Mixed feedback about web	
Partner organizations have positive feelings about the website	13
Partner organizations feel that the website needs improvement	5

Below is a full list of the partner organizations from which the sample we talked with was drawn.

Real Warriors Campaign Partner Organizations, as of July 2011

Adaptive Fly Fishing Institute
afterdeployment.org
Air Force Wounded Warrior Program
Alliant International University Continuing Education
Always A Soldier
America Supports You
American Foundation for Suicide Prevention
American Music Therapy Association
American Pain Foundation
American Psychological Association
American Red Cross
American Veterans with Brain Injuries
America's Heroes at Work
Anxiety Disorders Association of America
Arizona State University Virtual Counseling Center
Arlington Rotary Club
Armed Forces Foundation
Armed Services YMCA
Army Wife Network
Army Wounded Warrior Program
Association of the U.S. Army Family Programs

Blue Star Families
Blue Star Mothers of America
Brain Injury Association of America
Brain Trauma Foundation
BrainLine
BraveHeart: Welcome Back Veterans Southeast Initiative
California Department of Veterans Affairs
CBR YouthConnect
Cell Phones For Soldiers
Center for Deployment Psychology
Center for Telehealth and Technology
Center for the Study of Traumatic Stress
Challenge America
Citizen Soldier Support Program
Citizens United for Research in Epilepsy
Coalition for Iraq + Afghanistan Veterans
Comfort for America's Uniformed Services
Computer/Electronic Accommodations Program
Congressional Medal of Honor Society
Connect Veterans
Defense and Veterans Brain Injury Center
Defense Commissary Agency
Deployment Health Clinical Center
Disabled American Veterans
DoD Community Relations Directorate
DSTRESS Line
Educated Canines Assisting with Disabilities
Faith*Hope*Love*Charity
Family Resiliency Center
Fearless Nation PTSD Support
FOCUS: Families OverComing Under Stress
Folds of Honor Foundation
Fred Friendly Seminars
Freedom Is Not Free
Generations of Warriors Project
GI Film Festival
Give An Hour
Gold Star Wives of America
Grace After Fire
Hidden Wounds
Home Base Program
Home Front Hearts

Honor for All
Horses for Heroes/Professional Association of Therapeutic Horsemanship International
Horses Healing Heroes
Human Performance Resource Center
inTransition
Iraq Star
Jacob's Light Foundation
Joshua's Mission
Lest We Forget
Lone Star Veterans Association
Luke's Wings
Marine & Family Services–Marine Corps Community Services Henderson Hall
Marine Corps Combat Operational Stress Control
Mental Health America
Mental Health Association of Central Oklahoma
Military Child Education Coalition
Military Community and Family Policy
Military Officers Association of America
National Alliance on Mental Illness
National Alliance on Mental Illness Alabama
National Alliance on Mental Illness New Hampshire
National Alliance on Mental Illness Tennessee
National Association of State Head Injury Administrators
National Center for Telehealth and Technology
National Coalition for Homeless Veterans
National Football League Players Association
National Institute of Mental Health
National Intrepid Center of Excellence
National Military Family Association
Naval Center for Combat and Operational Stress Control
NCIRE - The Veterans Health Research Initiative
Not Alone
Operation Gratitude
Operation Helping Hands for Heroes
Operation Homefront
Operation Never Forgotten
Patriot PAWS Service Dogs
Pawsitive Perspectives Assistance Dogs
Pets for Patriots
Post-Deployment Health Reassessment–Army Support
Project New Hope Massachusetts
Project: Return to Work

Quantum Leap Farm
ReMIND/The Bob Woodruff Foundation
Reserve Officers Association
SAFE: Soldiers and Families Embraced
Semper Fi Fund
Sesame Workshop
Soldiers' Angels
Soldier's Heart
Sports Legacy Institute
Spouse READI
Stories That Heal Campaign
Strategic Outreach to Families of All Reservists
Strong Families Strong Forces
Student Veterans of America
Substance Abuse & Mental Health Services Administration
Talking with Heroes
Team Red, White and Blue
Tee it up for the Troops
The American Legion
The Brain Injury Recovery Network
The Coming Home Project
The Mission Continues
The National Center on Family Homelessness
The Satcher Health Leadership Institute at Morehouse School of Medicine
The Soldiers Project
The Wingman Project
There & Back Again
Tragedy Assistance Program for Survivors
United Services Organization
United States First Responders Association
United Through Reading
University of Colorado Depression Center
University of Michigan Depression Center
U.S. Department of Veterans Affairs
U.S. Department of Veterans Affairs OEF/OIF Outreach Teams
USA Cares
Veteran's Heart Georgia
Veterans Upward Bound
Virginia Wounded Warrior Program
Warrior Family Community Partnership
Warrior Gateway Program
What A Difference Campaign

Working Minds/Carson J. Spencer Foundation
Wounded Warrior Resource Center
Yellow Ribbon Reintegration Program
Zero to Three

APPENDIX E

Content Analysis Methods and Findings

To assess the content of the RWC campaign, we conducted a systematic review of the campaign's website, including all articles posted on the website, campaign dissemination materials, and video and radio public service announcements.

Content Analysis Methods

In May 2011, we reviewed and catalogued the content of the RWC website to gain a better understanding of the types of materials available. Materials were reviewed to identify the following information:

- Target population. The target population for each item reviewed was determined by the section of the website where the item was listed. Items applicable to additional populations were noted (e.g., article listed in the active duty section that may also be relevant for family members).
- Campaign goals. The materials were reviewed to determine which of the four campaign goals the materials supported: addressing the costs of inaction as compared with action, raising awareness of mental health services available, raising expectations of positive outcomes, and raising awareness of other resources.
- Purpose of the material. The materials were categorized as providing education or information, providing resources to promote help-seeking, or promoting the RWC (e.g., materials encouraging individuals to go to the RWC website).
- Whether the material included additional links to hotlines, other services or care, or additional information or education.
- If relevant, we also examined characteristics of individuals (i.e., gender, rank, race/ethnicity, branch of service) included in videos, PSAs, and pictures to assess the representativeness of the materials to the military population at large.

A single reviewer conducted the content analysis of all website material as of May 2011. The reviewer began by reading each material from beginning to end and then catalogued the target population, campaign goals, purpose of the material, whether the material contained additional links, and, if applicable, the characteristics of individuals. To ensure that the content analysis was consistently conducted by this single reviewer, a second reviewer also catalogued 10 percent of the content. Overall, the reviewers agreed as to the target population, campaign goals, purpose, additional materials, and representativeness of the content.

Reviewers agreed on 92.0 percent of the content measures. We also analyzed inter-rater reliability using a kappa statistic. The kappa statistic provides a normalized measure of agreement, adjusted for the agreement expected by chance. The kappa rating ranges from –1 to 1, where –1 is complete disagreement, 0 is agreement expected by chance, and 1 is complete agreement. The content-analysis reviews yielded a 0.79 kappa rating, which is considered indicative of substantial agreement (Landis and Koch, 1977). We did not find the kappa to be unduly affected by a relatively extreme percentage of raters consistently assuming positive ratings.

Findings from the Content Analysis

The RWC homepage is organized in such a way that campaign content is categorized and housed separately for different target populations and is easily accessible through a clearly marked link at the top of the website. Although most of the content falls within one of the five target populations, the campaign materials and videos, formerly housed together under the category "multimedia tools," were located in a separate area of the website. Because these items were grouped together at the time of the content analysis (June 2011), these materials were analyzed together and are represented by the heading "Multimedia Tools" in the analysis below. Of note, there are now separate links for campaign materials and videos on the RWC homepage.

Table E.1 displays the extent to which the content listed on a specific target population page (e.g., active duty, family) was relevant to, or aligned with, that target population and is based on a review of 49 multimedia tools, and articles targeting active duty (n=26), National Guard and Reserve (n=13), veterans (n=16), families (n=19), and health professionals (n=7). While in most cases the articles were relevant to the population under which they were listed, some content was also applicable to one or more additional populations but was not cross-listed.

Table E.2 describes the extent to which the articles listed for each target population aligned with campaign goals. As displayed in the table, the number of materials supporting each goal varied overall and within each target population. In addition, a significant number of materials also did not directly align with any of the campaign goals.

Table E.1
Real Warriors Campaign Website Content Alignment with Target Populations

	Content Is Relevant to the Target Population Under Which It Is Listed	Content Is Relevant to Another Target Population in Addition to or Instead of the Population Under Which It Is Listed	Content Is Not Relevant to a RWC Target Population
Multimedia tools	—[a]	—[a]	—[a]
Active duty	26	4	0
National Guard/Reserve	12	2	1
Veterans	15	0	1
Families	19	8	0
Health professionals	7	2	0

[a] These materials were not specifically directed at a single population.

Table E.2
Real Warriors Campaign Website Content Alignment with Campaign Goals

	Costs of Inaction Compared with Action	Awareness of Sign and Symptoms of Mental Health Problems	Raise Expectations of Positive Outcomes	Awareness of Services Available	Not Directly Relevant to Campaign Goals
Multimedia tools	6	21	26	29	9
Active duty	0	11	6	14	9
National Guard/Reserve	0	1	0	3	8
Veterans	0	3	4	4	9
Families	0	1	1	3	14
Health professionals	0	1	0	1	5

Campaign materials generally fulfilled one of three major purposes (Table E.3). First, many materials provided education or information on a range of topics relevant to mental health. Second, some materials were designed to promote help-seeking by providing, for example, information on where services could be obtained. A third purpose, promoting the RWC, included materials designed to promote the campaign or the website itself. Almost all of the materials in this last group were housed in the multimedia tools (now campaign materials) section of the website.

Given that most of the materials are relatively brief or provide higher-level summaries of a topic, we also examined the extent to which the materials provided links to additional information or services available for those who are ready to seek help. Most of these materials linked to additional information or education about the topic or to a hotline. Few provided direct links to mental health services (Table E.3).

A summary of findings from the content analysis is provided here.

Multimedia Tools. There were 49 multimedia tools available on the website, including brochures, posters, video and radio public service announcements, video profiles of warriors, and web banners. The majority of the tools were targeted toward active duty servicemembers. The populations represented were diverse and included male and female servicemembers; enlisted personnel and officers; white, black, and Latino servicemembers; and servicemembers from each branch of the military (excluding the Coast Guard). Most of the multimedia tools

Table E.3
Purpose of the Real Warriors Campaign Content by Target Population and Content Linkages to Additional Information or Services

	Purpose of the Content			Content Linkages		
Website Location	Education	Promote Help-Seeking	Promote RWC	Directly to Service Providers	Information/ Education	Mental Health Hotline/ RWC Hotline
Multimedia Tools	8	42	41	2	32	17
Active Duty	22	14	0	8	25	15
National Guard/Reserve	12	2	1	1	12	5
Veterans	13	6	0	3	15	8
Families	19	4	0	4	19	9
Health Professionals	7	2	0	1	8	1

addressed at least one campaign goal with a majority of the items raising awareness of available mental health services or raising expectations of positive outcomes. Only two of the items provided a direct link to services or mental health care, while 32 of the items provided links to additional information or education and 17 listed a phone number of a mental health hotline or the RWC hotline for additional support.

Active Duty. There were 26 articles and four resource link pages targeting active duty servicemembers. Resource link pages provide a listing of additional resources specific for that population. For active duty servicemembers, there are resource link pages for the Army, Navy, Marine Corps, and Air Force. For the purpose of the content analysis, we did not analyze the links provided on these pages. Of the articles, all 26 were directly applicable to active duty servicemembers, with five applicable to both active duty and another target population. Although the expert panel felt that the content of the articles on the website was most relevant for the Army and Marine Corps, among those articles with photographs, the majority depicted white, male, and enlisted servicemembers from all branches (excluding the Coast Guard). Only nine articles were not directly relevant to campaign goals. Fourteen articles raised awareness of mental health services. Additionally, most articles provided education about a topic or resources to promote help-seeking. Nearly all articles contained links to additional information or education and more than half listed the phone number of a mental health hotline, and eight articles provided a direct link to services or mental health care.

National Guard/Reserve. There were 13 articles and one resource link page targeting national guardsmen and reservists. Twelve of the articles were directly relevant to National Guard/Reserve, two were relevant to both National Guard/Reserve and another target population, and one article was not applicable to any target population. This article was written for civilian employers and provided tips for helping to ease the reintegration process of guardsmen and reserve servicemembers. Photographs in the articles featured mostly white, male servicemembers. Of the 13 articles, eight were unrelated to the campaign goals and three articles raised awareness of available services. Most articles provided education about a topic. Two articles provided resources to promote help-seeking and one article promoted the campaign itself. One article provided a direct link to a service provider and five listed the phone number of a mental health hotline.

Veterans. There were 16 articles and one resource link page targeting veterans. Fifteen articles were applicable to the veteran population and one article was not applicable to RWC population. That article listed things that the community can do to support veterans on Veterans Day. The photographs in the article represented male and female veterans who were either white or black, and represented the Air Force or Navy. Of the 16 articles, nine were not directly relevant to the campaign goals. The remaining articles served to raise awareness of mental health services and other resources and also to raise the expectations of positive outcomes. Most of the articles provided education about a specific topic and contained links to additional information or education. Three articles provided direct links to a service provider and eight listed the phone number of a mental health hotline.

Families. There were 19 articles and one resource link page targeting military families. All 19 were directly related to families, with eight also applicable to active duty servicemembers. All photographs in the articles showed male servicemembers representing three branches of service (Army, Air Force, Navy). The majority were white. Most of the articles, while relevant to mental health in general, were not directly related to the campaign goals. Of those that were, three raised awareness of mental health services and seven raised awareness of other resources.

All articles provided education about a topic and four also provided resources for help-seeking. All articles provided links to additional information, four linked directly to a service provider, and nine listed a phone number of a mental health hotline.

Health Professionals. There were seven articles and one resource page targeting health professionals. All articles were applicable to health professionals and two were also applicable to other populations. Four articles raised awareness of other resources and three were not directly applicable to campaign goals. Although related to mental health, these articles focused on becoming a TRICARE provider, understanding and using evidence-based clinical practice guidelines, and building resilience for military health professionals. Most of the articles provided education about a topic and two provided resources for help-seeking. Only one article linked directly to a service provider and listed the phone number of a mental health hotline, while all articles provided links to additional information.

Summary

The materials on the RWC website were targeted toward specific audiences and presented information for various communities including servicemembers, guardsmen and reservists, veterans, families, and health professionals. Though there are many resources available on the website, many are not directly relevant to the goals of the RWC. Excluding the multimedia tools and those specifically targeted at the active duty population, more than half of the material was not specifically relevant to the goals of the campaign. The campaign provides material relevant to its goals for the active duty population and for promotion of the campaign itself, but opportunities exist to improve the relevance of website materials for other populations relative to the RWC's goals.

Additionally, there are missed opportunities for information-sharing due to the lack of cross-referenced materials across target populations. Listing information in multiple places would not only increase readership but would also make the campaign website a more informative and useful tool for those seeking support or resources for mental health in the military community.

References

Adler, D. A., K. Possemato, et al. (2011). "Psychiatric status and work performance of veterans of Operations Enduring Freedom and Iraqi Freedom." *Psychiatric Services* **62**(1): 39–46.

Andreasen, A. R. (1994). "Social marketing: Definition and domain." *Journal of Marketing and Public Policy* **13**: 108–114.

Becker, M. H. (1974). *The Health Belief Model and Personal Health Behavior.* San Francisco: Society for Public Health Education.

Blazina, C., and L. I. Marks (2001). "College men's affective reactions to individual therapy, psychoeducational workshops, and men's support group brochures: The influence of gender-role conflict and power dynamics upon help-seeking attitudes." *Psychotherapy* **38**(3): 297–305.

Brady, K. T., T. K. Killeen, et al. (2000). "Comorbidity of psychiatric disorders and posttraumatic stress disorder." *Journal of Clinical Psychiatry* **61 Suppl** 7: 22–32.

Breslau, N., G. C. Davis, et al. (2003). "Posttraumatic stress disorder and the incidence of nicotine, alcohol, and other drug disorders in persons who have experienced trauma." *Archives of General Psychiatry* **60**(3): 289–294.

Britt, T. W., J. Davison, et al. (2004). "How leaders can influence the impact that stressors have on soldiers." *Military Medicine* **169**(7): 541–545.

Britt, T. W., T. M. Greene-Shortridge, et al. (2008). "Perceived stigma and barriers to care for psychological treatment: Implications for reactions to stressors in different contexts." *Journal of Social and Clinical Psychology* **27**(4): 317–335.

Cavanagh, J. T. O., A. J. Carson, et al. (2003). "Psychological autopsy studies of suicide: A systematic review." *Psychological Medicine* **33**(3): 395–405.

Coffman, J. (2002). *Public Communication Campaign Evaluation: An Environmental Scan of Challenges, Criticisms, Practice, and Opportunities.* Cambridge, MA: Harvard Family Research Project.

Coffman, J. (2004). *Strategic Communications Audits.* Washington, DC: Communications Consortium Media Center.

Corrigan, P., and B. Gelb (2006). "Three programs that use mass approaches to challenge the stigma of mental illness." *Psychiatric Services* **57**(3): 393–398.

Corrigan, P. W., J. D. Rafacz, et al. (2010). "Changing stigmatizing perceptions and recollections about mental illness: The effects of NAMI's in Our Own Voice." *Community Mental Health Journal* **46**(5): 517–522.

Corrigan, P. W., N. Rusch, D. Ben-Zeev, and T. Sher (in review). "Beyond the rational patient: Implications for treatment adherence and other health decisions." Manuscript submitted to *Social Science and Medicine.*

Defense Health Board Task Force on Mental Health (2007). *An Achievable Vision: Report of the Department of Defense Task Force on Mental Health June 2007.* Falls Church, VA: Defense Health Board.

Dertouzos, J., and S. Garber (2003). *Is Military Advertising Effective? An Estimation of Methodology and Applications to Recruiting in the 1980s and 90s.* Santa Monica, CA: RAND Corporation. As of February 22, 2012:
http://www.rand.org/pubs/monograph_reports/MR1591.html

Dertouzos, J., J. M. Polich, A. Bamezai, and T. W. Chesnutt (1989). *Recruiting Effects of Army Advertising.* Santa Monica, CA: RAND Corporation. As of February 22, 2012: http://www.rand.org/pubs/reports/R3577.html

Dickstein, B. D., D. S. Vogt, et al. (2010). "Targeting self-stigma in returning military personnel and veterans: A review of intervention strategies." *Military Psychology* **22**(2): 224–236.

Dorfman, L., J. Ervice, et al. (2002). *Voices for Change: A Taxonomy of Public Communications Campaigns and Their Evaluation Challenges.* Berkeley, CA: Berkeley Media Studies Group.

Dumenco, S. (2011). "How social media ranks fall TV's hit shows." *Advertising Age,* October 3.

Evans-Lacko, S., J. London, et al. (2010). "Evaluation of a brief anti-stigma campaign in Cambridge: Do short-term campaigns work?" *BMC Public Health* **10**: 339.

Faigin, D. A., and C. H. Stein (2008). "Comparing the effects of live and video-taped theatrical performance in decreasing stigmatization of people with serious mental illness." *Journal of Mental Health* **17**(6): 594–606.

Feldner, M. T., K. A. Babson, et al. (2007). "Smoking, traumatic event exposure, and post-traumatic stress: A critical review of the empirical literature." *Clinical Psychology Review* **27**(1): 14–45.

Fitch, K., S. J. Bernstein, et al. (2001). *The RAND/UCLA Appropriateness Method User's Manual.* Santa Monica, CA: RAND Corporation. As of February 22, 2012: http://www.rand.org/pubs/monograph_reports/MR1269.html

Glaser, B. G., and A. L. Strauss (1967). *The Discovery of Grounded Theory: Strategies for Qualitative Research.* Hawthorne, NY, Aldine de Gruyter.

Grant, B. F., F. S. Stinson, et al. (2004). "Prevalence and co-occurrence of substance use disorders and independent mood and anxiety disorders: Results from the National Epidemiologic Survey on Alcohol and Related Conditions." *Archives of General Psychiatry* **61**(8): 807–816.

Greene-Shortridge, T. M., T. W. Britt, et al. (2007). "The stigma of mental health problems in the military." *Military Medicine* **172**(2): 157–161.

Hammer, J. H., and D. L. Vogel (2010). "Men's help seeking for depression: The efficacy of a male-sensitive brochure about counseling." *The Counseling Psychologist* **38**(2): 296–313.

Henshaw, E., and Freedman-Doan, C. (2009). "Conceptualizing mental health care utilization using the Health Belief Model." *Clinical Psychology: Science and Practice* **16**(4): 420–439.

Hoge, C. W., C. Castro, S.Messer, D. McGurk, D. I. Cotting, and R. L. Koffman (2004). "Combat duty in Iraq and Afghanistan, mental health problems, and barriers to care." *N Engl J Med,* **351**: 13–22.

Independent Review Group on Rehabilitative Care and Administrative Processes at Walter Reed Army Medical Center and National Naval Medical Center (2007). *Rebuilding the Trust.*

Kessler, R. C., E. E. Walters, et al. (1998). "The social consequences of psychiatric disorders, III: Probability of marital stability." *American Journal of Psychiatry* **155**(8): 1092–1096.

Landis, J. R., and G. G. Koch (1977). "The measurement of observer agreement for categorical data." *Biometics* **33**(1): 59–174.

McFall, M., C. Malte, et al. (2000). "Effects of an outreach intervention on use of mental health services by veterans with posttraumatic stress disorder." *Psychiatric Services* **51**(3): 369–374.

National Institute of Mental Health (2010a). "NIMH Statistics: Major Depressive Disorder Among Adults." As of September 6, 2011: http://www.nimh.nih.gov/statistics/1MDD_ADULT.shtml

National Institute of Mental Health (2010b). "Post-Traumatic Stress Disorder Among Adults." As of September 6, 2011: http://www.nimh.nih.gov/statistics/1AD_PTSD_ADULT.shtml

Nielsen, J. (1994). *Usability Engineering.* San Diego, CA: Academic Press.

Noar, S. M. (2006). "A 10-year retrospective of research in health mass media campaigns: Where do we go from here?" *Journal of Health Communication* **11**(1): 21–42.

Office on Smoking and Health (2007). *Best Practices for Comprehensive Tobacco Control Programs–2007: Section A: Health Communications Interventions.* Atlanta, GA: U.S. Department of Health and Human Services, Centers for Disease Control and Prevention, National Center for Chronic Disease Prevention and Health Promotion.

Owens, G., C. Herrera, et al. (2009). "A preliminary investigation of mental health needs and barriers to mental health care for female veterans of Iraq and Afghanistan." *Traumatology* **15**(2): 31–37.

Pew Research Center (2011). *The Military-Civilian Gap: War and Sacrifice in the Post-9/11 Era.* Washington, DC. As of March 15, 2012:
http://www.pewsocialtrends.org/files/2011/10/veterans-report.pdf

Phillipson, L., S. Jones, et al. (2009). "Effective communication only part of the strategy needed to promote help-seeking of young people with mental health problems." *Social Marketing Quarterly* **15**(2): 50–62.

Pinfold, V. G., G. Thornicroft, et al. (2005). "Active ingredients in anti-stigma programmes in mental health." *International Review of Psychiatry* **17**(2): 123–131.

President's Commission on Care for America's Returning Wounded Warriors (2007). *Serve, Support, Simplify.* Washington, DC.

Rochlen, A. B., and W. D. H-oyer (2005). "Marketing mental health to men: Theoretical and practical considerations." *Journal of Clinical Psychology* **61**(6): 675–684.

Rochlen, A. B., R. A. McKelley, et al. (2006). "A preliminary examination of the 'Real Men. Real Depression' campaign." *Psychology of Men and Masculinity* **7**(1): 1–13.

Rochlen, A., M. Whilde, et al. (2005). "The Real Men. Real Depression campaign: Overview, theoretical implications, and research considerations." *Psychology of Men and Masculinity* **63**(3): 186–194.

Savoca, E., and R. Rosenheck (2000). "The civilian labor market experiences of Vietnam-era veterans: The influence of psychiatric disorders." *Journal of Mental Health Policy and Economics* **3**(4): 199–207.

Schnurr, P. P., A. F. Hayes, et al. (2006). "Longitudinal analysis of the relationship between symptoms and quality of life in veterans treated for posttraumatic stress disorder." *Journal of Consulting and Clinical Psychology* **74**(4): 707–713.

Seal, K. H., D. Bertenthal, et al. (2007). "Bringing the war back home: Mental health disorders among 103,788 US veterans returning from Iraq and Afghanistan seen at Department of Veterans Affairs facilities." *Archives of Internal Medicine* **167**(5): 476–482.

Smith, M. W., P. P. Schnurr, et al. (2005). "Employment outcomes and PTSD symptom severity." *Mental Health Services Research* **7**(2): 89–101.

Strauss, A. L., and J. M. Corbin (1998). *Basics of Qualitative Research: Techniques and Procedures for Developing Grounded Theory.* Thousand Oaks, CA: Sage Publications.

Tanielian, T., and L. H. Jaycox (2008). *Invisible Wounds of War: Psychological and Cognitive Injuries, Their Consequences, and Services to Assist Recovery.* Santa Monica, CA: RAND Corporation. As of February 22, 2012:
http://www.rand.org/pubs/monographs/MG720.html

Task Force on Returning Global War on Terror Heroes (2007). *Task Force Report to the President.*

Television Bureau of Advertising (2008). *2008 Media Comparisons Study.* New York, NY: Nielsen Media Research.

Vogt, D. (2011). "Mental health–related beliefs as a barrier to service use for military personnel and veterans: A review." *Psychiatric Services* **62**(2): 135–142.

Weinick, R. M., E. B. Beckjord, et al. (2011). *Programs Addressing Psychological Health and Care for Traumatic Brain Injury Among U.S. Military Servicemembers and Their Families.* Santa Monica, CA: RAND Corporation. As of February 22, 2012:
http://www.rand.org/pubs/technical_reports/TR950.html

Westphal, R. J. (2007). "Fleet leaders' attitudes about subordinates' use of mental health services." *Military Medicine* **172**(11): 1138–1143.

White House Office of National Drug Control Policy (2011). National Youth Anti-Drug Media Campaign. As of March 15, 2012:
http://www.whitehouse.gov/ondcp/anti-drug-media-campaign

Wulsin, L. R., G. E. Vaillant, et al. (1999). "A systematic review of the mortality of depression." *Psychosomatic Medicine* **61**(1): 6–17.

Zivin, K., A. S. Bohnert, et al. (2011). "Employment status of patients in the VA health system: Implications for mental health services." *Psychiatric Services* **62**(1): 35–38.